Disclaimer

The material in this book is presented for informational purposes only and not for the treatment or diagnosis of any disease. Please consult with a qualified health professional for any ailment discussed or mentioned herein. The author and publisher take no responsibility for the use or misuse of any information presented in this work.

Natural Q's: A Guide To Healthy Living

© 2004 by Timeless Voyager Press

ISBN 1-892264-16-1

TIMELESS VOYAGER PRESS
PO Box 6678
Santa Barbara, CA 93160

www.timelessvoyager.com

Covers and additional artwork editing: Bruce Stephen Holms
Photographer: Christa Havenhill
Illustrations: Jeff Yochim
Natural Q's is a Registered Trademark
Text © 2004 by Emil Faithe

Natural Q's

A Guide To Healthy Living

**Tips That Help You
Achieve Optimum Health**

Dr. Emil Faithe

Formatted by Bruce Stephen Holms

Edited by Linda White

TABLE OF CONTENTS

DEDICATION

This book is dedicated to my mom and dad, Sally and David Faithe, whose life-long struggle to find happiness and truth in the world has inspired me to do the same. This truth is for you. Your guidance and loving "cues" at every step of my life will never be forgotten.

ACKNOWLEDGEMENT

I wish to acknowledge with gratitude my partner and soul mate, Susan, for her never-ending love and support, without which, this book would not exist.

PREFACE

Many people are seeking to improve their health with vitamins, herbs, and other supplements these days. The problem is that there are so many supplements available from so many companies, all touting 'magical cures' for almost anything that ails you. What can we believe? Which supplements really are effective for what conditions? More importantly, which supplements are safe for you?

After years of observing the confusion, misinformation, and disappointment with self-treatment using supplements, I felt it was time to set the record straight.

This book is dedicated to those who are seeking the truth about how to nurture their bodies, and their spirit. It is my fondest desire that those who read this book will have a healthy and balanced understanding about what supplements, foods, and lifestyle choices help you achieve optimum health and well-being. This handbook will give you the 'Natural Q's' you've been searching for.

A Word From The Author

I am a pharmacist. Over my 22 years in practice I have dispensed thousands of different medicines for thousands of patients for hundreds of various ailments and maladies. I know that I have helped save the lives of many, and changed the lives of the rest. Daily, I pray that I have made a difference for all of them. Yet, all that said, I'm not sure what good I've really done. I've always felt that even though I was being paid well to do this job, being a pill pusher wasn't exactly what I had in mind for my life's work.

I remember clearly thinking, in June of 1981, when they smiled, shook my hand, and presented me with my doctorate certificate in pharmacy, that I was going to do something different with my career, and my life. This was not going to be your standard "lick 'em and stick 'em" (a coined phrase for putting labels on prescription bottles) medicine man. No way.

It took a while, as all good things do, however, and in the summer of 1993, she stepped up to the prescription counter. Sadly, I don't even recall her name. But it could have been anyone… nameless, faceless, man or woman. She handed me stack of eight new prescriptions. I checked the computer. She was already taking ten other prescriptions. I looked her in the eye, and boldly asked "are you feeling any better"? She thought about it for a moment, then replied "No, not really".

Here was a woman, in her early fifties, in the so-called prime of her life, spending hundreds of dollars each month on prescriptions, seeing a half dozen doctors, enduring the nagging side effects of a dozen or so prescriptions, and she was no better than the day she started on her healing journey years earlier.

It was like a huge slap in the face for me... the wake up call I had been waiting for. And even though this particular day, this particular woman inspired my new path as a natural medicine man, I had personally seen and heard of hundreds of other cases that were strikingly similar. People weren't getting any better, despite the honest intent of countless doctors who intervened on their behalf.

My life as natural healer and teacher, and this book, is the result of that experience.

Dr. Emil Faithe

Dr. Faithe resides in Phoenix, Arizona where he maintains a natural health and life guidance practice. For questions or consultation appointments, you may contact Dr. Faithe by email: <drfaithe@life-guide.com>.

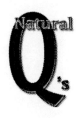

Natural Q's

Everyone is looking for ways to stay healthy these days. For this reason, and many more, the dietary supplement industry, those involved with the sale of vitamins, herbs, and other supplements, or what I will call 'Natural Medicines', is enjoying incredible popularity.

Everyone is selling something natural to keep you healthy. There's an overabundance of products to buy, and even more places to buy them. The internet, grocery store, and even the local gas station seem to be selling natural medicines. I recently went to fill up my car with gas. As I started to pay the cashier, a young woman about 17 years old, I spotted a display of packets of the herb ginkgo biloba at the checkout counter. I think many would agree that the Chevron station is not the ideal place to make important health choices, especially with the particularly potent natural medicine, ginkgo biloba. The point is that natural medicines are all too readily available for purchase by anybody, from anybody, for any reason. And this can be dangerous. We should be prudent when it comes to making choices about our health. We should ask questions, and more importantly, seek answers. We should make every effort to recognize what is happening to our minds and our bodies. That said, I urge you to sense, watch for, and listen to those Natural Q's that are all around us. Here are a few tips for you to consider as you make choices about how to feed yourself and care for yourself in a healthy fashion. These tips are what I refer to as Natural Q's for healthy living:

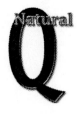 # Natural Doesn't Necessarily Mean Healthy

First, understand that just because something is natural doesn't mean it's good for you.

And what does 'natural' mean, anyway? Arsenic is a natural product. It comes from the earth. I wouldn't recommend consuming any of that. Poison ivy, too, is a plant that comes from the earth. Isn't that 'natural'? We need to be sensible and realistic about what we consider 'natural'. We need to use good judgement.

Your body knows what it wants. If it doesn't like what you're putting in it, believe me, it will let you know. The problem is that most people don't really pay much attention to what their body is trying to tell them. However, if we listen carefully, pay close attention to those subtle sounds, pangs, pains, changes, and 'feelings', if we just stop long enough to give our body the patience and respect it deserves, we can make sensible, healthy choices.

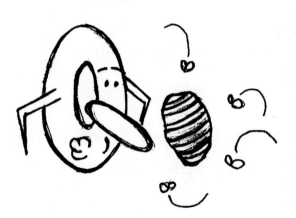

Listen to your body's
Natural Q's.

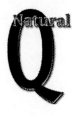 # Natural Medicines Are Drugs

By definition, natural medicines change the way the body works.

They alter the effects of certain specific pathways and mechanisms in our body. This can result in the development of side effects, and increase the risk for interactions with prescription medications, as well as other natural medicines. We should treat natural medicines with the same respect we treat prescription medicines. You wouldn't buy $130.00 worth (a one month's supply) of the prescription ulcer medicine Prevacid and start taking it without any guidance, no more than you would you buy a set of blueprints to build a house without some knowledge of how to build it.

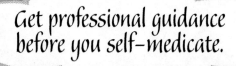

Get professional guidance before you self-medicate.

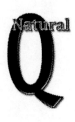 # Most People Who Take Natural Medicines, Take Too Many

Most people I see in my practice take altogether too many natural medicines.

Many use products they don't need, products that are duplicates, unnecessary, expensive, or that can actually make them feel worse rather than better. Why? Because there's too much information out there, much of it skewed to sell products, much of it incomplete, or just plain inaccurate. My advice is to avoid becoming emotionally attached to everything you read or hear about natural medicines.

Everybody has an opinion about what natural medicine can cure this or can make you look like that. They want you to believe how safe their product is, how quickly it works, how powerful it is, how you can't live without it, and so on. Perhaps you recall hearing those radio ads that shout at you: "Lose 10 pounds in just 3 days, or your money back." Sound familiar? HOLD ON! More is not better. Faster is not better. The human body doesn't understand 'fast'. Stay clear of these kinds of offers.

Does your body (not your mind) really want to lose 10 pounds in 3 days? Do you really want to grow your hair back with a product that contains a dozen different herbs that could interact with your blood pressure medication or your blood thinner? Probably not. And that's a smart call.

Natural medicines are, for the most part, unregulated by the FDA. Anyone can pretty much sell whatever they want and say just about anything, and THEY DO. My advice? Buyer Beware.

> *Take only the natural medicines that you need with guidance from a practitioner you know and trust.*

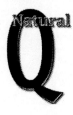

Buy Quality Products

Buy your natural medicines from a large, reputable company that has something to lose; otherwise, they may not care if you lose.

Ask about the quality assurance measures they use to check the purity and potency of the products they sell. Invariably, at about this time in my seminars, the question pops up: "So, Dr. Faithe, which brands do you recommend?" At the risk of being incomplete or biased, I will merely say, there are a number of reputable, seasoned natural medicine manufacturers who sell quality products to health care practitioners, health food stores, and other outlets. If you have a specific question in this regard, please reach me directly at my office.

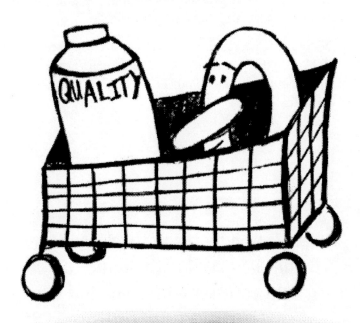

Get guidance if you're not sure.

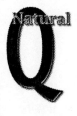

Natural Medicines Have Side Effects And Interactions

Natural medicines DO interact with prescription medicines, and they DO sometimes have 'side effects'.

In both cases, these can be mild, severe, or even life-threatening. In general, however, they tend to be less common and less severe than with prescription medicines. Natural medicines can also interact with other natural medicines, and even certain foods and medical conditions.

The lesson is actually quite straightforward. Yes, it may be convenient to pick up a head of lettuce, then grab a bottle of the herb kava for your nerves (because the kids are screaming to buy those sugar-filled cookies). However, kava can cause liver problems, especially with that bottle of wine you're buying for dinner or that Tylenol for your tension headache. Take time to learn more about what you're about to put into your body.

Learn more about what you put into your body!

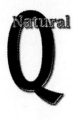

Don't Stop Your Prescriptions Without Guidance

It's always advisable not to stop any prescription medicines without consulting the doctor who wrote that particular prescription.

There are several reasons for this. First, there can be withdrawal reactions by stopping a prescription medicine suddenly. Second, the medicine prescribed for you could be crucial to keeping your heart beating correctly or to keeping some other vital organ working correctly. Finally, it's important (and courteous) to keep your doctor in the health care loop.

> It's important to keep your doctor in the health care loop.

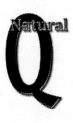

Natural Medicines Should Not Always Replace Your Prescription Medicines

In most cases, I recommend that you don't just stop taking your prescription medicines cold turkey and replace them with natural medicines.

Natural medicines should, at least initially, be ADDED, or integrated into your existing prescription regimen to help improve your condition even further.

As symptoms improve with the use of natural medicines, your doctor should be consulted to discuss the possibility of decreasing the doses of certain medicines, and then, if possible, the prescription medicine may be eliminated entirely. It is a process. Be patient!

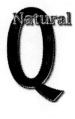 # You're In Charge Of Your Body

Many patients tell me, "I would never tell my doctor that I take supplements.

He would be angry with me." Many report that their doctor doesn't believe in, or worse yet, 'pooh poohs' anything 'natural'. Comments like "there are no studies" or "we don't know if they're safe" or "they're not FDA approved" are often heard from some doctors. Don't blame your doctor for not knowing about natural medicines. If, however, they don't want to know about natural medicines and you do, ask them to recommend or refer you to someone who is a natural medicine expert. If they can't or won't, just check the yellow pages under 'holistic practitioners'.

Oh, by the way. All decisions about your body, your health, your life...are yours. You call the shots. If you're not in agreement with what your doctor tells you, if you don't see eye-to-eye, shop around.

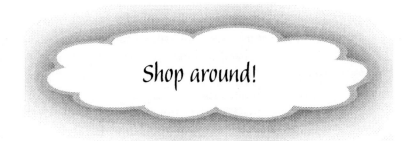

Shop around!

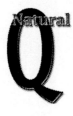 # Watch For 'Baby Steps'

Natural medicines work more slowly than prescription medicines, but for many people, they DO work.

Often, we see 'baby steps' in improvement, and the only way we can see that a natural medicine is working is to stop it for a while and assess how you feel. And remember, just like prescription medicines, some natural medicines work for some people and not for others. Be patient, and be realistic in your expectations. That way, you'll never be disappointed.

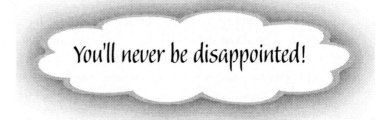

You'll never be disappointed!

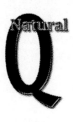 # Your Most Important Medicine Is Food

Your best natural medicine is FOOD. Food is the foundation of healthy living.

Food provides the fuel to keep our bodies running efficiently, and for a long time. In some cases, however, the amount of nutrients we need to improve a specific medical condition are not practically available in any food. A good example is the natural medicine glucosamine. You'd have to eat a whole lot of crab shells to get nearly enough of the active ingredient chitin to improve the symptoms of your arthritis.

Nonetheless, there's healing power in foods. And only when we can't eat enough foods to get all the healing ingredients, and only then, do we supplement with natural medicines. That's why they call them 'dietary supplements'. Natural medicines are a supplement to healthy eating, and healthy living.

Making conscious choices to eat the right foods can make all the difference in the quality, and quantity, of life. Remember that the foods you eat can either heal you, or they can harm you. Learn more about healthy food choices in the "Food Q's" chapter.

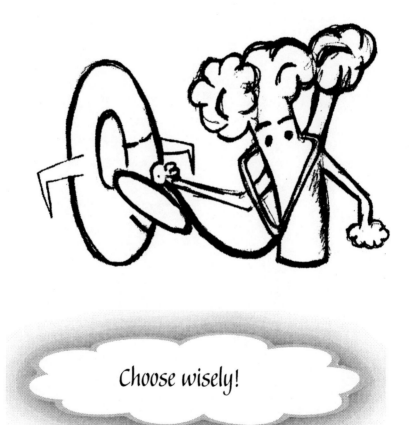

Choose wisely!

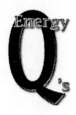

Energy Q's

Now, many of you are going to read this chapter with the idea that I'm going to tell you how to improve your energy, or vitality, naturally.

Not so. I'm going to talk about energy of a different color, or current. Yes, you can improve your energy and strength naturally, and perhaps you'll pick up a pointer or two about that somewhere in this book. The energy I'm referring to, for lack of a better term, is the natural electric energy field that makes up the human body and pulsates through all of our cells, tissues, and organs. Some would refer to this as the life energy force, or the like.

The body is comprised of fields of energy flowing from within our center, creating an AURA, or a shield of energy around us. The body is all energy. I realize that this concept may be difficult to visualize. Let me simplify matters. In a healthy body, all energy moves freely and easily, flowing to all areas of the body in perfect balance. When this energy flow becomes unbalanced or does not flow smoothly or freely through all areas, it can become blocked or 'stuck'. When energy gets stuck, we create an environment or opportunity for illness or disease.

Let It Flow And Let It Go

I couldn't mean this more literally. Let it go!

When we become angry, fearful, or resentful, no matter what the cause; when we don't resolve these situations and release these feelings, energies become blocked. Depending on where this energy becomes blocked, or stuck, can determine the kind of disease we get.

One of my patients came to see me with a serious case of rheumatoid arthritis in her hands. After I reviewed her natural medicines, we had a nice discussion, as I always do, about when, how, and what may have been the root cause of these symptoms. She proceeded to tell me that she had been fighting the State over some land rights for a number of years, and that this had been causing her to be angry and resentful. She had been 'holding on' to what she believed to be her rights. As it turns out, her arthritic symptoms began shortly after her intense and consuming battle with the State began.

High blood pressure, or hypertension, affects over 50 million Americans. In many cases this condition can be the result of "holding in" (not releasing) anger, frustration, resentment that is created in our daily lives. As an example, a woman in her late fifties came to me to discuss her blood pressure and the heart problems she had developed over the past few years. She admitted to having long-standing relationship conflicts with her

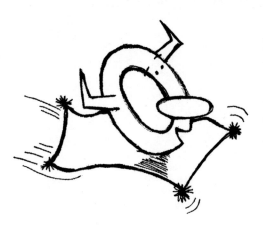

sibling, whom she truly admired. The energy in her heart area had stagnated, facilitating the development of her heart dis-ease. I can cite hundreds of similar stories, all with the same motto.

Let it go!!!

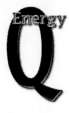

You Can Do It Yourself

Many illnesses can be prevented, even cured, if these blockages are prevented or re-opened in time.

So, how do you release these blocks? It's really quite simple. You can do it yourself without any intervention from the science of medicine: Let go of the negative emotions and thought patterns that are controlling your life.

Let's face it. We've all had negative thoughts and feelings from time-to-time. And it's easy to blame these feelings and emotions on everything else in our lives, our jobs, our spouse, bad luck, or whatever. Many of us hold on to these negative patterns because we've become attached to them; they form a comfort zone and become a way of life. . .or maybe, no life.

Each of us has the power to change all that, to resolve our feelings of anger, resentment, and fear. And when you do, you open the door for healing to take place, AND you may just find that your long-standing symptoms have lessened, or even gone away.

Sounds great! Where do I start?

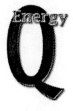

Forgive Yourself

It all starts with you. Forgive yourself for anything you believe you may have unjustly done to yourself.

Realize that you are a perfect being just as you are. Yes, you may want to have more money, lose weight, get that dream job. You can. You deserve perfect health and a fulfilling life. Know this.

Forgive yourself, believe in yourself, and go for it. I believe you'll find that the nicer you treat yourself, the better you'll feel. The better you feel, the more often you'll smile. And that's good.

> The nicer you treat yourself,
> the better you'll feel!

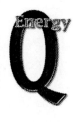

Forgive Others

We've all been slighted or mistreated by someone, somewhere down the line. It's a part of life's lessons.

And some may feel like they've had more than their fair share of hurt, whether it be emotional, physical, financial, or otherwise. Forgive those who have treated you unjustly. Yes, at first the anger and resentment toward these people may seem insurmountable, even unforgivable. But it can be done.

I saw a patient in my office with crippling arthritis in her hands. She could hardly move her fingers, and this was particularly devastating because she was a watercolor painter. It turns out that she had been harboring a longstanding grudge against her elderly mother whom she now felt obligated to care for. Yes, I

31

started her on some glucosamine, but we saw even greater improvement in her symptoms by exposing the source of her anger and resentment and performing release exercises. Soon after, she found herself able to move her fingers more freely and began painting once again.

It may take a little time to completely forgive, or it may be immediate. Either way, start the process today. Forgive THEM because it's good for YOU. You just may notice that when you forgive others, your emotional, physical, and financial health will start improving. You'll feel better, and the better you feel, the more often you'll smile. And that's good.

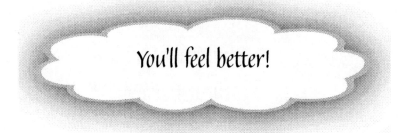

You'll feel better!

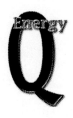

Stop And Take Inventory Of Your Life

Most of us go through life accepting our unhappiness and our less-than-optimal health and well-being.

Oddly enough, we relinquish control of these intimate and important facets of our lives to others rather than take responsibility for them ourselves. Many people believe that psychologists and medical doctors should direct our health and happiness. I disagree. We are all capable of having a positive impact on our health and happiness if we would just slow down enough to see how we got where we are. Why do you have joint pain? Why are your blood sugars so high? Why did you become depressed? How did you come to be thirty pounds overweight?

Take an inventory of your life. All of it. Look at the events that have transpired in your life and take a look at your life now. Figure out what led you down this path to your present day, to your present state, and take sound, calculated steps to turn it around. If you're unable to do it yourself, seek professional assistance from someone who understands the concepts of personal energy release and balancing, or contact my office.

Are you packing away unresolved, anger, resentment, fear, or other issues deep down inside? Deal with these issues and live a more fulfilling and happy life. You deserve it.

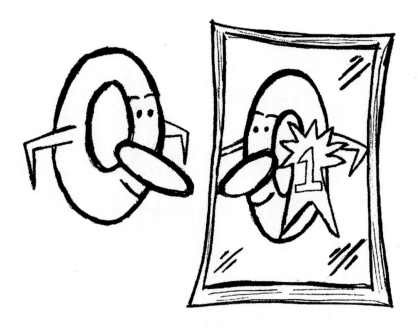

Live a more fulfilling and happy life.

Life can be more fulfilling and joyful
when you forgive and release.

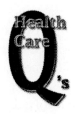

Health Care Q's

Health Care has come a long way, baby. Less than 100 years ago there were very few prescription medicines, and there were no health care conglomerates.

There weren't any urologists, cardiologists, oncologists, anesthesiologists, pediatricians, or pulmonologists. If you needed to see a doctor, that meant you were really sick. There was one doctor, often working out of a small office without any assistants, and he knew all about you, and your family. He, or she, probably delivered you from the womb, along with the rest of your siblings, and when it came time to take care of the bill, there were no insurance cards to process or papers to fill out. You paid cash, or, in some cases, bartered the fee.

Today, health care is 'managed' by systems, computers, and lots of people, most of whom don't know who you are and have absolutely nothing to do with making you feel better. In many cases, more time is spent updating your insurance information than is spent in the entire visit with your doctor.

The health care system in the United States makes it too easy, almost 'tempting' to see a doctor for even the most minor ailment. That's because it seems like such a good deal to be able to pay only $10 or $20, or in some cases nothing, to see a doctor for any reason. Some people tend to visit doctors unnecessarily, sometimes just to have someone listen or pay attention to them. Frequent doctor visits, however, do not necessarily mean better health. On the contrary. More visits with more different doctors can complicate your health care. See your doctor when you need to, not when you don't.

Over the years I have found that many of my patients were dissatisfied with their doctor visits. In many cases, they were feeling no better; in some cases, they were feeling worse. Then there's the myriad of prescription medicines and procedures that were tried and failed, or caused side effects, not to mention the time and expense involved.

Then there is the big issue of having more than one doctor taking care of you. One for your sinuses, one for your knee pain, one for your breathing problems, and so on. Often, these doctor's offices, despite their best efforts, were not coordinating your care or talking to each other as often as needed. The result: many patients failed to see results. It's at this point that many patients seek out 'alternative', 'complimentary', or holistic practitioners to help them heal. Now, that's not to say that allopathic doctor's don't do good work. In many cases, the health care system gets in the way of quality care.

Given all that, when should you schedule a visit with your doctor? Here are several Natural Q's to help make your decision a little easier:

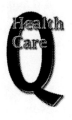

Do All That You Can To Take Good Care Of Number One (That's You)

It seems like the logical thing to do. However, as a society, it seems that we have generally relinquished all responsibility for the care of ourselves to someone else. Take back control and responsibility for your health. Start by doing all the right things for yourself:

Eat right (see "Food Q's")
Exercise regularly (see "Exercise Q's")
Clear your mind (meditate) (see "Inside Q's")
Take appropriate supplements when necessary

If you're doing all the right things (and your body will tell you if you're not), and if things still don't feel right, schedule a visit with a doctor.

And although Western medicine doctors may be covered by your 'plan', keep an open mind. Perhaps a natural pharmacist, nutritionist, acupuncturist, chiropractor, Reiki practitioner, or other holistic or complimentary practitioner who is NOT on your plan may be right for your condition. In fact, paying out-of-pocket to see someone who's NOT on your plan, may be 'cheaper' in the long run.

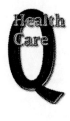

Prepare For Your Office Visit

Be prepared to answer specific questions about the condition that brings you to the office to begin with. Make notations as to when the symptom(s) started, how long they last, exactly where it bothers you, what time(s) of day it occurs, if you've ever had this happen before, etc.

By all means, always tell your doctor about all the medicines you are taking, including the vitamins, herbs, and protein shakes, and anything else you put into or onto your body. I recommend actually bringing in the bottles of everything you are taking to your office visit. Even though some doctors may be less than enthusiastic to see your suitcase full of vitamins, ask them to make notations in your record of all of them.

Be prepared to discuss the types and quantities of food you eat, as well as any other pertinent lifestyle issues like alcohol consumption, tobacco use, caffeine use, etc.

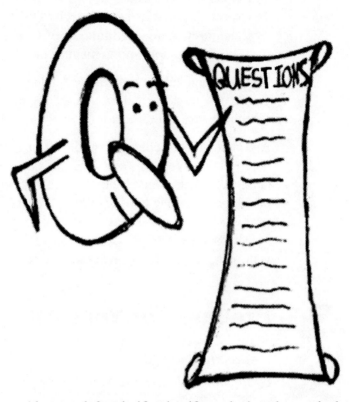

Always ask for clarification if you don't understand what is being said. Whenever your MD, PharmD, ND, DOM, or other practitioner writes a prescription or recommends a therapy, whether that be in the form of a technique, an exercise, or a pill, ask the following questions (and do be polite and respectful at all times):

• What is this?

• How does it work?

• How will I know if it's working for me?

• How long will I have to take/do this?

• Are there any side effects, or ill effects?

• What do I do if these effects occur?

• How do I take it/do it? (with food, on an empty stomach?)

Tell your doctor if you are extra sensitive to medicines. Inform them of your blood type, either O, A, B. If you don't know your blood type, ask the doctor to 'type' your blood the next time you need a blood test. Blood types can influence not only the types of foods that are right for you but even the types of medical conditions you are prone to.

Finally, and this is a keeper, you don't have to agree with everything they recommend. You may know some things about your system, yourself, about your constitution, that they do not. In fact, you often do. If you feel uncomfortable with a recommendation, a test, a pill, a procedure, tell them so. Ask if there are any other ways to achieve the desired results. Perhaps there are alternative medicines, modalities, even other practitioners, that you might try first.

It's important to have honest, open communication with the people who are helping you take care of your health. It's also important to remember who's in charge of your body. You are.

Remember who's in charge of your body.

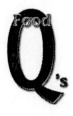

The Food Q's

It all starts with food-the fuel that makes us go and keeps us healthy. The type of fuel we burn determines how well our machine runs.

Spend time researching what kinds of fuel your body really needs. It's actually easier than you might think. That's because your body will eventually tell you if it doesn't like what you're feeding it. And different bodies can have different preferences, often dependent on blood type, body type, genetics, lifestyles, and more.

What are some of the signs that your body doesn't like what you're feeding it? You might **gain weight, experience indigestion, stomach cramps, muscle cramps, gas, constipation, diarrhea, headaches,** and even **allergic reactions** ranging from **skin rashes** to **respiratory collapse**. Our body is always giving us signs. It knows what fuels it prefers. We just need to listen carefully.

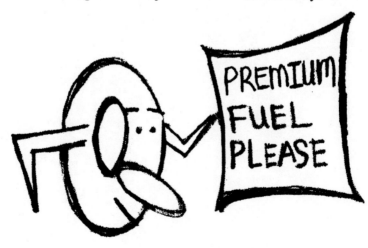

Let's review the basics once again. The foods you eat can either heal you by sustaining healthy cell functioning and growth, or they can harm you by opening the doors for altered, unhealthy cell growth. Here's the message: Choose your foods carefully. Here are some 'Q's' to help you along the way:

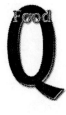

Avoid Unnatural Food Additives

This includes MSG, aspartame, AKA (Nutrasweet, Sweet'N Low), artificial colors, flavors, preservatives, etc.

Even the seemingly healthy salad bars often use sulfites to preserve the fruits and vegetables. Many people experience headaches as well as blood pressure and respiratory problems when they consume sulfites. Wine also contains naturally occurring or added sulfites to keep the product from spoiling.

Read the labels of everything you put in, and on, your body (including the 'inactive' ingredients). Buy and cook with organic, free-range, pesticide-free, and chemical-free products whenever possible, and try to eat at restaurants who boast the same.

These food additives, and others, have been implicated as the cause of many of our chronic diseases.

> Food additives can cause
> chronic disease.

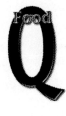

Cook With Cast Iron Or Stainless Steel Cookware

There are concerns that aluminum cookware, even Teflon-coated aluminum, may be implicated in excess aluminum accumulation in our bodies, possibly contributing to Alzheimer's and other diseases.

Choose pure cast iron or stainless steel cookware and cutlery when you have the choice. And all choices are yours.

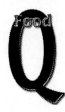

Eat Your Fruits And Veggies

Yes, an apple a day can keep the doctor away. And a couple servings of broccoli a day could keep the oncologist (cancer specialist) away.

That's because broccoli and other greens contain natural immune stimulants and anticancer ingredients. Besides all that, vegetables are an ideal source of fiber, and they contain generous amounts of calcium. Diabetics would do well to maximize their vegetable fiber, since fiber can lower blood sugar, cholesterol levels, and more.

Lot's of people complain that veggies cause a lot of gas. Broccoli, cabbage, and others can be the culprit. That's because they contain sulfur components. Use a broad spectrum, vegetable-based, digestive enzyme to help reduce this problem. Take 1 dose with the first bite of these veggies.

When you make your vegetable choices, minimize the amount of corn you consume since corn can upset the digestive tract and trigger allergic reactions. Carrots are healthy eating but they contain a fair amount of sugar. Diabetics should enjoy carrots, but not in excess.

> *Vegetables and fruits for good health.*

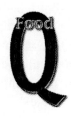

Limit Dairy, Alcohol, Sugars, Animal Protein

Let's talk about cow's milk.

The concern is that it comes from cows, and that means it contains a high amount of cow (bovine) protein, which may not be compatible with every human's immune system. Lactose intolerance is but another reason for limiting cow's milk and other dairy products.

Consider using rice milk (my favorite) or soy milk, if you're not allergic to soy (and many people are.) Nut and grain milks are also available, such as almond milk, oat milk, and others. Sure, these milks taste different than cow's milk, but you can become accustomed to it. And let's face it, the first time you tasted cow's milk you had to get used to that taste, too, if you can remember that far back.

One last note on cow's milk... contrary to popular TV commercials, it's not the only dietary source of calcium. Eat your veggies!

Alcohol in the form of beer, wine, and even distilled spirits probably does decrease the risk of heart disease but should be used in moderation.

Liver problems, mood disturbances, and triglyceride elevations are some of the less desirable effects of alcohol consumption. Alcohol can cause problems when combined with prescription medicines that cause drowsiness, like the antianxiety medicines (Xanax, Ativan, etc.), the antidepressants (Paxil, Zoloft, etc.), and others. Alcohol also interacts with a number of natural medicines like kava, St. John's wort, to name a few.

Sugar. It tastes great, but it can cause mood disturbances, especially in children.

Many people crave this tasty carbohydrate, but once the rush is over, many people tend to become moody and irritable. Try to limit your consumption of these simple carbohydrates (like cookies, crackers, breads, and pastas) that are loaded with sugar, and stick with the complex carbohydrates in your vegetables. Eat your veggies!

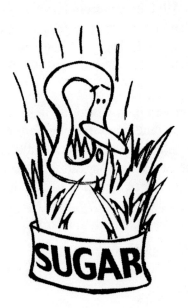

FYI, people who suffer from ADHD, including little people, fare substantially better when dairy and sugar is eliminated from the diet.

Lean red meat can be healthy; however, an excess of animal protein has been implicated as the cause of a number of chronic diseases, including osteoporosis.

Now, I'm not suggesting that we all become strict vegetarians. That's a matter of personal choice. If you choose to consume animal protein, stay with free-range, pesticide, and chemical-free meats where possible. If you enjoy your burgers and steaks, don't deprive yourself. Enjoy them in moderation. Everything in moderation.

This a good time for me to remind you of this very important point: Don't attempt to turn your diet, or your life, inside out all at once. That's a recipe for failure. If you enjoy Boston cream pie, filet mignon, and Krispy Kreme doughnuts, make your changes gradually, one at time. And you don't necessarily have to give up everything completely. Just cut back on portion sizes and frequency of consumption, when and where you can. And remember: Be good to yourself.

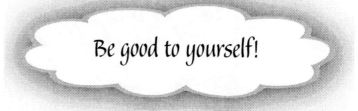

Be good to yourself!

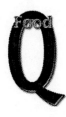

Eat Plenty Of Whole Grains

Include brown rice, beans, nuts, mushrooms, onion, and garlic.

These foods are loaded with nutrients, antioxidants, and plenty of fiber. Use organically grown sources whenever you are able.

Whole brown rice may have cancer preventative properties, and mushrooms and onions are great for the immune system, as well. There's lots of evidence that garlic can help reduce cholesterol and blood pressure, and it has powerful antifungal, antiviral, antibacterial activity, to boot.

A good rule of thumb is this: if you can grow it or catch it, it's probably good for you. Just make sure it's free of harmful pesticides and other chemicals. The moral of this story: Minimize the amount of packaged and processed foods you eat.

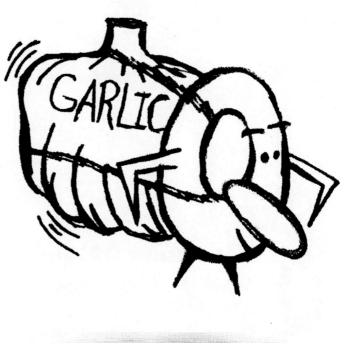

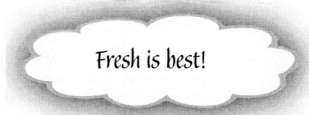

Fresh is best!

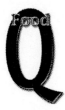

Cook With Healthy Oils

Cooking with olive oil is a great way to help reduce cholesterol levels, and it's been shown to reduce the incidence of colon cancer, as well.

Cook with oils that are low in saturated fats and high in polyunsaturated fats. Remember that flax seed oil is a healthy choice to add to anything, but you can't cook with it. Getting it hot denatures the important fatty acids.

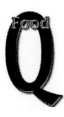

Read The Labels On All Food Products

When all else fails, read the labels.

This is your best assurance that you're getting everything you expect. Unfortunately, the labeling laws are quite lenient, and sometimes less than desirable additives will be listed, or disguised as a different or unfamiliar name. If you're not sure what's on the label or in the food product, contact the manufacturer.

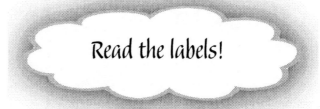

Read the labels!

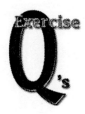

The Exercise Q's

A lot of people make a career of teaching other people how to exercise.

Thousands of books have been written on the subject by some of the most renowned experts in the field. Rather than comment on all that conventional wisdom, let's talk basics.

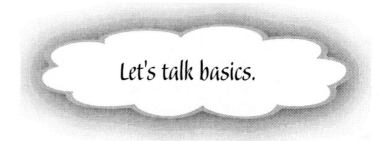

Let's talk basics.

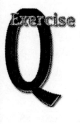

It's Not How Long And Hard You Exercise, Just Get Some On A Regular Basis

Our bodies need exercise on a regular basis to maintain tip- top condition, and there are a number of ways to get it.

The gym is a great place to get guidance on building specific muscle groups, and you can even run on the treadmills there, if you please. It can also be a nice social event for those who are so inclined. If you choose to get your exercise at the gym, and it works for you, continue it.

However, what I have found over the years is that many people simply don't want to leave their home, get in a car, and go to a 'place' to get exercise. It takes too much time, too much effort, and sometimes too much money to get started.

Getting the exercise that fits your lifestyle doesn't have to be complicated or expensive. For many, the key to success is developing a routine, a regimen that fits into your day on a regular basis. So where do you start?

Walking is a great form of exercise. And you don't have to do power walks.

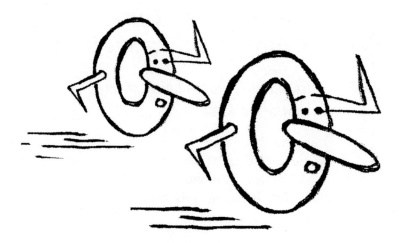

Even if you simply 'stroll' around your neighborhood 4 to 6 times a week, you can improve your mood, your energy, and reduce the risk of osteoporosis and other conditions. Work up to 30 to 45 minutes each time you walk, and work at a pace that is comfortable to you.

If you have arthritis or other painful conditions, or carry excess weight, just start slowly and go at your own pace. Even if you can only walk 5 feet the first day, that's great! Work up slowly to the distance that's comfortable for you. If you suffer from painful conditions that limit your movement, glucosamine, MSM, or the high potency enzymes taken on an empty stomach can make a big difference. If your doctor has limited your activity due to a medical condition, by all means, follow his/her advice.

Walking is a great form of exercise!

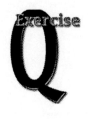

Take Care Of Your Cardiovascular System

Many people enjoy running several miles a day, every day of the week.

Over time, this can be hard on the joints. Even more important, the cardiovascular system can become inflamed; that is, the blood vessels can become swollen. Recent studies warn that this kind of inflammation of the cardiovascular system over periods of time can increase the risk of heart attacks. If you enjoy long distance running or other intense, continuous exercise, consider adding a high potency enzyme to help reduce the inflammation.

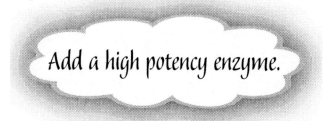

Add a high potency enzyme.

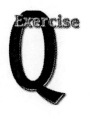

Maintain Healthy Exercise Hygiene

Avoid exercising close to bedtime hours since this can stimulate many organ systems, making it difficult to sleep at night. Of course, drink plenty of fluids, consume a healthy diet, and be careful not to do either in excess just before your work out.

Those who are in training, or 'working out', often use protein shakes and carbohydrate drinks to help build muscle mass. These supplements can be safe and effective for many people. But take my advice: stay clear of all steroid or steroid like products, as well as creatine. These products can be dangerous when used incorrectly or for long periods of time, and the results are usually temporary. Be natural!

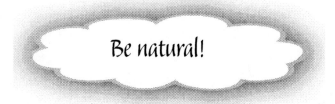

Be natural!

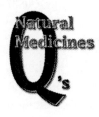 # Natural Medicines Q's

One of the most important things to understand about natural medicines is that they can, and do, interact with prescription medicines and other natural medicines, and these interactions are real.

Some of these interactions are important since they have a real possibility of occurring and/or causing you harm. Others are less important and are either less likely to occur, or if they do occur, they are generally mild.

The more prescription medicines you take, the greater the chance of an interaction. If you take prescription

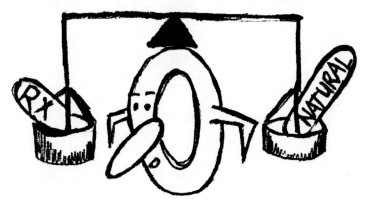

medicines or over-the-counter medicines on a regular basis, consult with a natural medicine expert before you start your natural regimen.

As a rule, herbs tend to have more interactions than vitamins, minerals, or other supplements. A classic example is the herb St. John's wort. St. John's wort has no less than a dozen important interactions, several of which can be dangerous if not monitored (see St. John's wort monograph).

One of the most important interactions that can occur with natural medicines, are those that affect the thickness, or viscosity of the blood. When you use blood-thinning natural medicines in combination with prescription or over-the-counter medicines that can also thin the blood, bruising or bleeding becomes a real concern. Although often mentioned, bruising or bleeding rarely occurs, but when it does, it should not be ignored. Bruising tends to precede bleeding, but not always. Pay close attention to bleeding from any site or any changes in energy levels.

If you are prone to blood clots, or if you have any other blood problems, pay extra attention to all the medicines you take, including natural medicines.

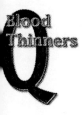

Prescription & OTC Blood Thinners

*Here's a list of just some of the common prescription and over-the-counter (OTC) medicines that have a tendency to cause blood thinning. These medicines, when combined with one or more natural blood thinners, **may** cause the blood to thin too much:*

Prescription & OTC Blood Thinners	
• Coumadin	• Vioxx
• Aspirin	• Celebrex
• Motrin	• Plavix
• Naprosyn	• Ticlid
• Aleve	

The prescription blood thinner Coumadin interacts with many prescription medicines as well as many natural medicines. It is always a 'red flag' when you are contemplating self-treatment with natural medicines. However, this does not mean that you absolutely can never take ginkgo or garlic or other blood modifying natural medicines. What it does mean is that you should:

1. Get professional guidance on how to dose and use the natural medicine before you start

2. Tell your doctor(s) about all natural medicines you are taking

3. Tell the lab tech that draws your blood about all natural medicines you are taking

4. Be alert for bruising or bleeding

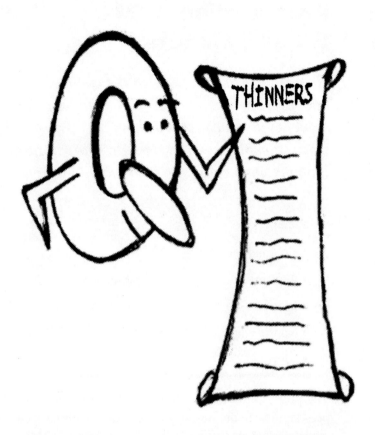

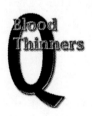

The Natural Blood Thinners

Here is a list of just some of the most common ones: If you're not sure about your natural medicines, contact my office for more information.

Natural Blood Thinners	
• Aloe Vera	• Evening Primrose Oil
• Chondroitin	• Feverfew
• Dong Quai	• Fish Oil
• Flax Seed Oil	• Garlic

Natural Blood Thinners	
• Ginger	• Ginseng
• Ginkgo Biloba	• Green Foods
• MSM	• Vitamin E

Several natural medicines can also THICKEN the blood and work against Coumadin. Two of the most common are Co-Enzyme Q10 and St. John's wort. If you have a clotting disorder or take Coumadin, get advice before you start either of these natural medicines.

I have been asked many times about what natural medicines could be used as a substitute for Coumadin. First, there is no true natural substitute for Coumadin. Despite that fact, many people have opted to keep their blood thin by combining several natural medicines on a regular basis. Although this may prove to be effective for some conditions and for some people, there is no assurance that clotting will not occur, and there is no reliable way to measure the effectiveness of this practice. On the other hand, this natural blood-thinning regimen may have protective effects. If you choose this option, consult with a natural medicine expert before you start, and do let your primary doctor know what you're doing.

Consult with a natural medicine expert.

The Side Effect Q's

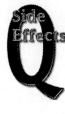

Natural medicines can cause side effects.

These side effects tend to be less severe and less troublesome than with prescription medicines, but they can occur. The most common side effect you may experience with natural medicines is gastrointestinal (GI) upset. This may include cramps, bloating, diarrhea, gas, nausea, etc. Headaches or rashes may also occur. In many cases, these unwanted effects will lessen over the first few days of therapy. If they do not, we need to determine which natural medicine is causing the problem and either reduce the dose or try something different.

Everyone reacts to medicines differently. A natural medicine like flax seed oil, for example, may suit one person just fine. However, another person may experience cramping and loose bowels. The same holds true for prescription medicines. If you are extra sensitive to the effects of prescription medicines, you are likely to be extra sensitive to the effects of natural medicines. Make sure to tell your practitioner if you are extra sensitive to natural medicines.

Most side effects occur within the first few doses of the medicine while some may appear as much as days to weeks down the road. Side effects can often be minimized by starting with lower doses and working slowly up to higher doses.

As with all medicines, if you experience a side effect, discontinue the likely culprit until the symptom subsides. Your natural medicine practitioner can help you do an 'elimination' regimen to weed out the problem medicine.

Allergies to natural medicines are also possible. Again, this is more common with herbs than with vitamins, minerals, or other supplements. For example, the herbal immune stimulant echinacea comes from the ragweed, or daisy, family. So does the liver-protective herb, milk thistle, and others. If you're allergic to daisies, you may experience an allergic reaction to either one of these herbs. These reactions can range form an itchy skin rash, to breathing problems, all the way to full respiratory collapse.

Yes, natural medicines tend to have less frequent and less severe side effects than prescriptions, but it's wise to maintain a healthy respect for them. After all, they are drugs.

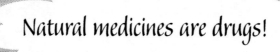

Natural medicines are drugs!

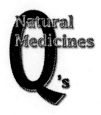 # The Dosing Q's

How To Take, And Not To Take, Natural Medicines

After years of working with people and their natural medicines, I've learned a number of important things. Here's something I'd like you to remember: Most people who take natural medicines take too many of them.

Most people who take natural medicines take too many!

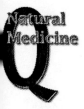

Don't Take More Medicine Than You Need

Please take my advice. More is not better.

Take only the natural medicines that you need for the specific condition or symptom you want to improve. No more than that. (This holds true for prescription medicines, too.)

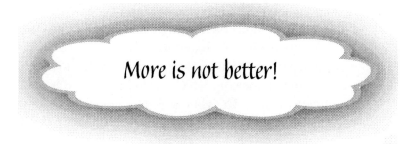

More is not better!

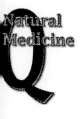

Give Your Body A Vacation From Supplements

Give your natural medicines a break now and then.

What I recommend to my patients, and now to you, is to stop all supplements on the weekend. Give your liver a chance to clear everything out. Drink extra fluids over the weekend to help your liver with this task, then resume your regimen on Monday. Some people may complain that they need to take certain natural medicines 7 days a week to keep their pain level down or to keep their digestive system functioning, etc. That's fine. Just stop as many as you can on the weekends.

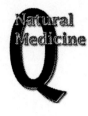

Most Supplements Should Be Taken With Food

The question is often asked about which natural medicines to take on an empty stomach and which ones to take with food. Some people become very concerned and confused about when to take them, and in their struggle to get it just right may miss some doses altogether. So let me put your mind at ease.

There are very few natural medicines that must be taken on an empty stomach to be effective, and even if you took them with food, it wouldn't be tragic. Some medicines just work better on an empty stomach. Examples of this are SAM-e, aloe vera, and acidophilus. Many people find it helpful to write out a little schedule indicating which medicines should be taken at which time of day. Do your best to remember how to take your medicines, but don't spend too much time or thought on how to juggle those pill bottles.

> Remember how to take
> your medicines.

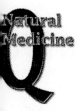

Take Each Dose With A Big Glass Of Water

This goes for your prescription medicines, too.

Take all medicines with at least 8 ounces of water, preferably 1 medicine at a time. Avoid swallowing a handful all at one sitting. This is often too much for the stomach and intestine to absorb, plus taking everything all at once may cause GI upset.

Take all medicines with water.

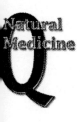

Natural Medicines Work Slowly (and that's good)

I'm often asked: "How do I know if these natural medicines are actually working?" The answer? Stop taking them for a while and see how you feel.

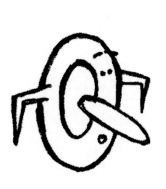

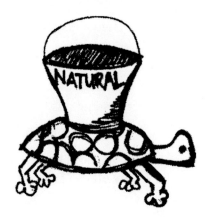

Because natural works more slowly and gently than prescription medicines (and that's the way the body prefers it), you often don't notice how far you've improved until you stop taking them. Try it some time. Stop one of your supplements for a week to 10 days and make a note about how you feel. You can always restart at any time. If you're taking St. John's wort, don't stop suddenly (see St. John's wort monograph).

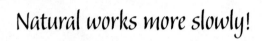

Natural works more slowly!

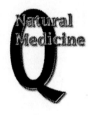

Natural Medicines Can Help Keep You Healthy

If you don't have any medical conditions, do you still need to be taking any kind of natural medicine supplementation?

Not everybody needs to supplement with natural medicines; however, many people find improved energy, vitality, and overall health when they follow a good basic regimen. Here's my suggested regimen for healthy humans who wish to stay healthy:

• High potency multiple vitamin with high B complex

• Calcium/Magnesium

• Flax seed oil

• Acidophilus

• Digestive enzyme

If you need further guidance on specific doses or brands, contact my office. Here's to your health!

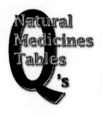

The Natural Medicines Tables

Just a few Q's before we start.

1. Many of the natural medicines listed here have similar or overlapping uses. This doesn't mean you should try all of them at the same time. Start with one medicine, and give it time to work.

2. Not all possible or potential uses are listed, nor does any medicine necessarily work for all listed uses, or for all people.

3. Unless otherwise specified, the doses listed are for healthy adults. Consult your practitioner for doses for any other age groups or medical conditions, or contact my office for further guidance.

4. This information is not a substitute for good clinical judgment from a qualified practitioner. If you don't feel well, seek the advice of a qualified medical practitioner.

5. If you're uncertain about how to use any natural medicine, or if you have any acute condition, including pain, fever, or any kind of injury, always seek the advice of a qualified practitioner. Do not self-treat.

6. If you take prescription medicines, get guidance from a natural medicine expert before you begin using any natural medicines.

7. None of the medicines listed here are intended to treat, cure, or diagnose any medical condition (Sorry, I'm required to say that).

TABLE 1: Acidophilus

Natural Medicine	Acidophilus
Use:	candida, cold sores, diarrhea, food allergies, GERD, immune stimulant, irritable bowel syndrome, lactose intolerance
Side Effects:	Acidophilus may cause gas.
Drug Interaction:	Acidophilus may be inactivated when taken at the same time as an antibiotic dose. Take acidophilus at least 2 hours before or after any antibiotic.
Supplement Interaction:	No significant supplement interactions.
Dosage:	The dose you take will depend on the specific product you purchase. Acidophilus comes as a capsule, liquid, and powder, and in various strains and potencies. Use the recommended dose 1/2 hour before meals every day, and stay with it continuously.

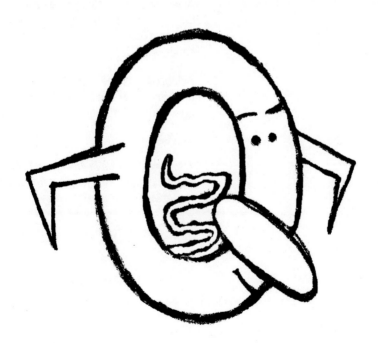

Natural Medicine	Acidophilus
Comments:	Acidophilus is the *friendly bacteria* that can thwart pathogenic or *unfriendly bacteria*, thereby reducing the number and severity of infections.
	Although commonly referred to as 'acidophilus', there are various other strains of probiotics, or 'friendly bacteria', one of which is Lactobacillus Acidophilus. Others include Lactobacillus GG, Lactobacillus Bulgaricus, Bifidobacterium Bifidum, and others. Some of the best 'acidophilus' products will contain up to 8 different strains.
	Store acidophilus in the refrigerator to maintain potency.
	I am often asked if eating yogurt is a good way to get these bacteria. Yes, but often we need more than is available in yogurt alone.
	Acidophilus can help reduce excess estrogen levels in women, reducing the risk of breast cancer and other hormone-related cancers.
	Acidophilus is one of those natural medicines that can be beneficial at every age, and on a continuous basis.
Cost Factor:	$10-$25
Natural Q:	*Using acidophilus in infants and children can help reduce the number and severity of ear infections, and respiratory infections.*

TABLE 2: Aloe Vera Juice

Natural Medicine	Aloe Vera Juice
Use:	arthritis, autoimmune disorders, cancer, candida, chronic fatigue syndrome, constipation, colitis, diabetes, fibromyalgia, irritable bowel
Side Effects:	Diarrhea, stomach cramping, and palpitations can occur.
Drug Interaction:	Aloe may interact with digoxin and other heart medicines that regulate your heart beat. Since aloe may reduce your potassium levels, get guidance if you're taking potassium supplements or diuretics ('water pills').
Supplement Interaction:	Aloe may interact with hawthorn or other herbs used to stimulate the heart. Use with licorice may reduce potassium levels even further. Aloe may interact with other laxative stimulant herbs like senna leaves.
Dosage:	Start with 1 to 2 tablespoonsful of 99.7% pure product aloe vera juice once or twice daily, at least 1/2 hour before food, and gradually work up to 3 to 4 times daily. You'll know you're taking too much when you get watery stools, in which case you should reduce to the next lowest dose.
Comments:	Aloe should not be used on a routine, long-term basis, since it may lead to laxative dependence.
	Diabetics should monitor their blood sugars carefully since aloe vera can lower blood sugars.
	Aloe vera juice may be more effective than capsules. Aloe vera juice should be stored in the refrigerator once opened.
Cost Factor:	$10-$20

Natural Medicine	Aloe Vera Juice
Natural Q:	*Aloe vera gel used on the skin is excellent for burns, wound healing, even pre-cancerous skin lesions.*

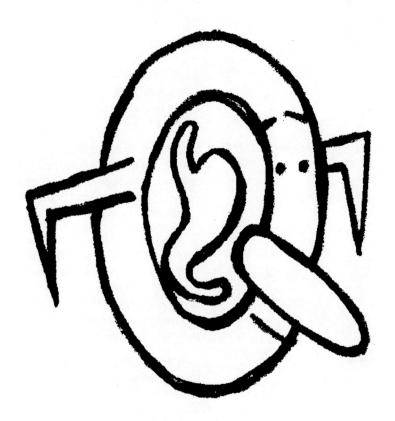

TABLE 3: B-Complex Vitamin

Natural Medicine	B-Complex Vitamins
Use:	acne, anxiety, carpal tunnel syndrome, depression, energy, hair growth, liver support, menopausal symptoms, migraines, neuropathies, PMS, restless legs syndrome, skin conditions
Side Effects:	Stomach cramping, nausea, skin flushing, itching, and headache can occur with the B vitamins.
Drug Interaction:	Vitamin B6 (pyridoxine) may reduce the effect of certain Parkinson's medications.
Supplement Interaction:	No significant supplement interactions.
Dosage:	Start with a complex that contains 25 to 100mg of vitamin B1, B2, B3, B6. Don't exceed 300mg of vitamin B6 (pyridoxine) per day, since this may cause neurological problems. B complex products often contain other B, or B-like vitamins such as vitamin B5 (pantothenic acid), vitamin B12 (cyanocobalamin), folic acid, choline, inositol. Always take B vitamins with food.
Comments:	Women using oral birth control are often vitamin B deficient.
	B vitamins may turn urine yellow-orange.
	B vitamins work best in combination, although additional amounts of any B vitamin can be added for specific conditions.
	Vitamin B12 is especially helpful in Alzheimer's patients and in older people with depression. It is often used under the tongue (sublingually) in the form of tablets or liquid. Sublingual formulations may cause a 'rush' or 'flushing' reactions.
Cost Factor:	$10-$20

Natural Medicine	B-Complex Vitamins
Natural Q:	*The B vitamins can be very useful in improving mood, energy, and more, especially in the elderly.*

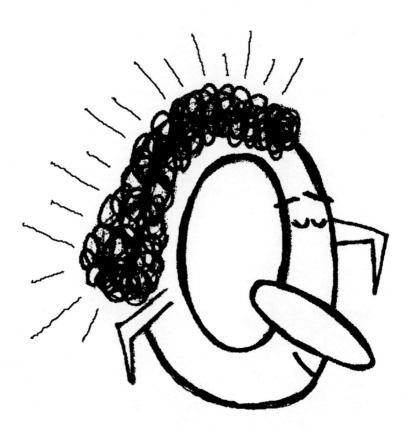

TABLE 4: Black Cohosh

Natural Medicine	Black Cohosh
Use:	hot flashes, menopausal symptoms, painful menstruation
Side Effects:	May cause stomach cramping, nausea, or headache. Some women are extra-sensitive to black cohosh and may experience muscle aches, nervousness, weakness, or blood pressure changes.
Drug Interaction:	No significant drug interactions.
Supplement Interaction:	No significant supplement interactions.
Dosage:	Start with 20mg once daily with food and stay with it for 30 days. If the response is not adequate, use 20mg twice daily and stay with it for 3 months. If you're substituting this medicine for Premarin, taper the Premarin slowly once black cohosh is started.

Natural Medicine	Black Cohosh
Comments:	Black cohosh has estrogenic-like activity and has been shown to improve bone density and protect against heart disease like prescription estrogens, without the increased risk of cancer and other negative effects.
	Don't confuse BLACK cohosh with BLUE cohosh, which is used for uterine stimulation.
	The question often arises, "Can I use black cohosh if I'm still taking my Premarin?" It's probably safe, but why do both?
	Some women require hormone level testing to help determine which hormones need balancing. I prefer saliva hormone sampling for improved accuracy.
	Consume lots of legumes, such as soy beans, garbanzo beans, and green beans to get natural plant estrogens from food.
Cost Factor:	$10
Natural Q:	*Black cohosh can improve the symptoms of arthritis.*

TABLE 5: Calcium

Natural Medicine	Calcium
Use:	diarrhea, hypertension, osteoporosis, restless legs syndrome
Side Effects:	Gas can occur in some cases. Calcium can cause constipation, and for those who suffer from diarrhea, this can be good. This is also one of the reasons calcium supplementation should be 'buddied up' with magnesium supplementation. Don't take either one long term without the other. They work well together.
Drug Interaction:	In theory, calcium supplementation can reduce the effect of the medicines known as the calcium channel blockers, such as Norvasc, Cardizem, Verapamil, and others, potentially reducing their effect. Calcium might also reduce the effect thyroid hormones, tetracycline, and the fluoroquinolone antibiotics like Cipro, Levaquin, etc. This can be minimized by taking calcium 3 to 4 hours before or after taking these medications.
Supplement Interaction:	No significant supplement interactions.
Dosage:	In general, use calcium doses of 500 to 1500mg daily in 2 to 3 divided doses with food. Postmenopausal women need doses closer to 1500mg daily to help reduce osteoporosis. Remember that cow's milk is not the only dietary source of calcium. Green leafy vegetables as well as other greens, seafood, oats, and almonds are also a substantial, and preferable, source.

Natural Medicine	Calcium

Comments:

Make sure you take at least 400 units of vitamin D daily to help improve calcium absorption.

There's been controversy regarding the use of calcium supplements and the development of kidney stones. Many studies indicate that calcium from FOOD sources actually is more responsible for this problem than calcium supplements.

Should you separate your calcium from your magnesium dose? It's nice if you can, but really, I'm not concerned in the least if they're taken at the same time.

I'm often asked: "What's the best kind of calcium to take?" There are many good ones including calcium citrate, maleate, chelates, and hydroxyapatite. Calcium carbonate isn't 'bad', and it does contain more calcium per dose than the others, but because it tends to lower stomach acid, it's not well absorbed. Calcium carbonate blended with other calcium forms is a good call.

Calcium in combination with magnesium can help reduce blood pressure and the nagging restless leg syndrome many experience when they sleep.

Cost Factor: $10

Natural Q: *Calcium supplementation can reduce the incidence of colorectal cancer.*

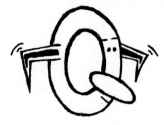

TABLE 6: Co-EnzymeQ10

Natural Medicine	Co-EnzymeQ10 (CoQ10)
Use:	angina, congestive heart failure, diabetes energy, hypertension, immune stimulant, migraines, muscular dystrophy, Parkinson's, respiratory conditions
Side Effects:	CoQ10 may cause GI upset, and for some people, heart palpitations.
Drug Interaction:	CoQ10 may thicken the blood, reducing the effect of the blood thinner Coumadin.
Supplement Interaction:	No significant supplement interactions.
Dosage:	Start with 50mg daily and work up to 300mg daily in divided doses, with a fatty meal. Doses up to 600mg per day or more are sometimes used. Get guidance from your practitioner before going that high.
Comments:	Consider taking CoQ10 if you take the prescription medicines known as the beta blockers (Tenormin, Lopressor, etc.), the 'statins' used to lower cholesterol (Mevacor, Zocor, Lipitor, etc.), or glyburide, since these medicines deplete CoQ10 levels in our bodies. CoQ10 can be used to reverse the toxicity of the cancer medicine Adriamycin. CoQ10 formulated in the liquid-filled soft gelatin capsules may be more effective, and I prefer them.
Cost Factor:	$30
Natural Q:	*CoQ10 rubbed onto the gums twice daily can improve periodontal disease.*

Co-EnzymeQ10

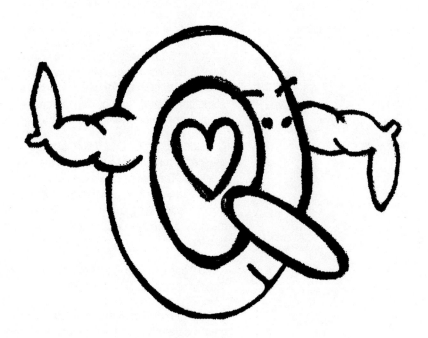

TABLE 7: Digestive Enzymes

Natural Medicine	Digestive Enzymes
Use:	candida, food allergies, gas, GERD, heart disease, irritable bowel syndrome, lactose intolerance, pain , Parkinson's
Side Effects:	Digestive enzymes can cause GI upset, even possible bleeding. Avoid them if you have bleeding disorders, or if you have active ulcers.
Drug Interaction:	If you're taking prescription blood thinners like Coumadin, aspirin, or ibuprofen, monitor for bruising or bleeding.
Supplement Interaction:	If you take natural blood thinners, monitor for bruising or bleeding.
Dosage:	Take 1 tablet or capsule with your first bite of regular, full-size meals. Don't use with smaller meals or snacks. For improving heart disease and pain, use the ultra-high potency enzyme combination products on an empty stomach 2 to 3 times daily. Depending on the brand you use, take 1 to 6 tablets per dose and work up slowly. Always take enzymes, and all medicines, with at least 8 ounces of water to keep them from sticking to your esophagus.

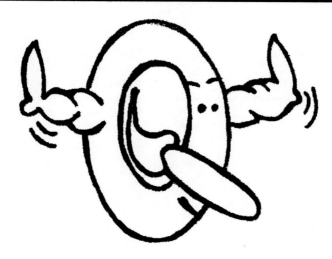

Natural Medicine	Digestive Enzymes
Comments:	COMMENTS:

COMMENTS:

There are many enzyme combinations available. At a minimum they should contain lipase, amylase, protease, and ideally lactase, bromelain, and papain. Some may contain trypsin, chymotrypsin, and other ingredients.

Although the papaya enzyme alone can help with digestion, for some it is not enough. Eating papaya or pineapple (the source of bromelain) can also be helpful.

Contrary to popular medical thinking, reducing the production of acid with medicines like Pepcid, Prilosec, and Prevacid, etc. can leave food undigested in the stomach, actually worsening GERD and heartburn. Adding a broad-spectrum enzyme can actually improve these symptoms, and more.

Enzymes can reduce the inflammation of the cardiovascular system, thereby reducing the incidence of heart attacks and possibly stroke. They can also reduce the pain and inflammation of arthritis and other painful inflammatory conditions.

Cost Factor: $20

Natural Q: *Diabetics can benefit from digestive enzymes because enzymes can break down carbohydrates more completely.*

TABLE 8: Echinacea

Natural Medicine	Echinacea
Use:	antiviral for cold and flu, immune booster, topically, for wound healing
Side Effects:	People who are blood type O may notice muscle or joint aches when using echinacea. If you suffer from autoimmune disorders like lupus, multiple sclerosis, rheumatoid arthritis, HIV, and others, you may experience an increase in the symptoms associated with these diseases. Nausea and skin rash are possible with echinacea, especially if you are allergy prone.
Drug Interaction:	If you take prescription medicines like prednisone, methotrexate, cyclosporine, etc. to lower your immune system, echinacea can reduce their activity. Use with caution.
Supplement Interaction:	No significant supplement interactions.
Dosage:	There are dozens of brands of echinacea available in capsule and liquid formulations, and in various dosages. Follow the directions on the package. I often recommend dosing up to 4 to 6 times daily at the first sign of cold or flu for the first 1 to 2 days, reduce to 3 to 4 times daily, and continue until the symptoms are resolved, plus about 3 days, then stop. Don't use echinacea year round. Echinacea can be used in children ages 4 and up at lower doses.

Natural Medicine	Echinacea
Comments:	Echinacea is part of the ragweed, or daisy, family. If you are allergic to ragweed, stay clear of echinacea. It may cause skin rashes, asthma, even anaphylaxis. Many people use echinacea in combination with goldenseal or other immune stimulants. If you suffer from upper respiratory, urinary tract, or GI tract infection, this combination makes sense. If not, use echinacea alone. Make sure not to use this goldenseal/echinacea combination for more than 10 days straight since goldenseal can harm your liver over periods of time.
Cost Factor:	$10
Natural Q:	*Echinacea salves and poultices can help heal many kinds of skin wounds or lesions.*

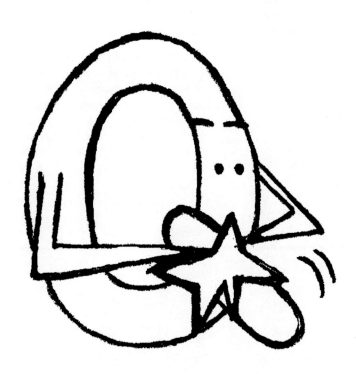

TABLE 9: Fish Oil

Natural Medicine	Fish Oil
Use:	ADHD, arthritis, asthma, bipolar disease, chronic fatigue syndrome, colitis, coronary artery disease, depression, eczema, fibromyalgia, high cholesterol, hypertension, lupus, Reynaud's syndrome
Side Effects:	Fish oils are noted for causing 'fish belching' or having a fishy taste. They can also cause nausea. This is reduced when taken in the middle of a meal. Liquid fish oil, available in packets, seems to cause less belching.
Drug Interaction:	Higher doses of fish oil can cause bruising or bleeding, especially when combined with Coumadin, Plavix, aspirin, Motrin, etc.
Supplement Interaction:	Fish oils may increase the possibility of bruising and bleeding when combined with natural medicines that thin the blood.
Dosage:	Fish oil is often referred to by its 2 main active ingredients: EPA (eicosapentaenoic acid) and DHA (docosahexanoic acid) which can come in various concentrations, depending on the product. I recommend dosing by total grams of fish oil, from the fish body, to avoid confusion. For most conditions, start with 1 gram twice daily taken in the middle of meals. Work up slowly to 2 grams twice daily. Bipolar disease and other conditions may require doses up to 10 grams per day. Work up to these doses gradually.

Natural Medicine	Fish Oil
Comments:	Like the other natural oils, fish oils are a very versatile natural medicine. Cod liver oil has similar activity to the fish body oils, but may contain higher amounts of vitamin A and D, which can accumulate in our bodies. Using a combination of fish and flax seed oil is often quite effective in improving the symptoms of ADHD and bipolar disease over a period of 3 to 4 months. Fish oil may be very useful for improving psoriasis.
Cost Factor:	$10-$20
Natural Q:	*Eat fish 3 to 4 times weekly to help maintain good health. Salmon, mackerel, and tuna are good choices.*

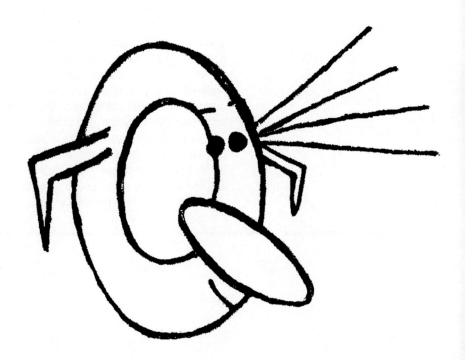

TABLE 10: Flax Seed Oil

Natural Medicine	Flax Seed Oil
Use:	ADHD, arthritis, autoimmune disorders, cancer, chronic fatigue syndrome, cholesterol , constipation, coronary artery disease, depression, hormone balancing, immune stimulant, irritable bowel syndrome, lupus, memory, multiple sclerosis, skin conditions
Side Effects:	Flax seed oil may cause loose stools or gas.
Drug Interaction:	Flax seed oil, like all oils, can thin the blood. Monitor for bruising or bleeding when used with Coumadin, aspirin, Motrin, etc.
Supplement Interaction:	Flax seed oil may thin the blood. Used in combination with other natural medicine blood thinners it may cause bruising or bleeding for some people.
Dosage:	Take 1 to 2 tablespoonsful daily with meals. Mix with yogurt, cottage cheese, or any beverage to disguise the taste. Many describe the taste as 'nutty and oily'. Just stir and drink quickly. Adding flax seed oil to your protein shakes is another convenient way to disguise the taste. Many people enjoy their flax seed oil straight. For those who don't, the capsules work fine. Just remember the conversion factor: 14 (fourteen) capsules equal 1 tablespoonful of liquid.

Natural Medicine	Flax Seed Oil

Comments:

This is a very versatile and effective natural medicine, and one of my favorites. Flax seed oil contains the omega 3, 6, and 9 fatty acids that are important for many bodily functions.

Refrigerate both the capsule and liquid forms, and watch expiration dates. Like all oils, flax seed oil has a limited shelf life, and fresh is best. Shake the liquid well before using.

I'm often asked if flax meal added to cereals offers similar efficacy. It won't hurt to add the flax meal, but I recommend using these pressed oils along with the flax meal to get the maximum effect.

Cost Factor: $10-$20

Natural Q: *Flax seed oil is an excellent choice for chronic fatigue syndrome and fibromyalgia.*

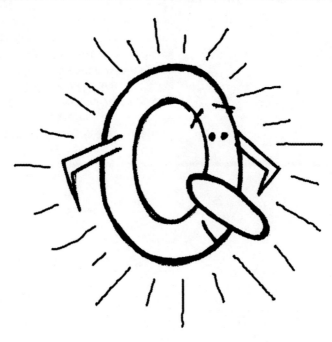

TABLE 11: Garlic

Natural Medicine	Garlic
Use:	antibacterial, antifungal, antiviral, candida, cholesterol, hypertension, immune stimulant
Side Effects:	Garlic may cause GI upset, including gas. There is no true 'odor-free' garlic, and mouth and skin odors are common. Only the mouth odor is reduced with the enteric-coated tablets. Garlic will be excreted through the skin.
Drug Interaction:	Garlic may thin the blood. Use with caution when combined with blood-thinning medicines like Coumadin.
Supplement Interaction:	Garlic may provide additional blood thinning when combined with natural medicine blood thinners.
Dosage:	Dosing garlic can be tricky, since it's prepared and labeled in various ways, depending on the manufacturers. The active ingredient is the odorous allicin component; however, garlic doses are often expressed as milligrams of fresh garlic. Use 600 to 900mg daily with food, or follow the directions on the label. Stay with the enteric-coated tablets. If you wish to consume fresh garlic, 1 clove daily is a reasonable dose. Just warn your friends.

Natural Medicine	Garlic
Comments:	Controversy exists as to whether 'aged' or 'fresh' garlic supplements are best. Studies indicate that 'fresh' garlic supplements have more activity per dose, and those are the ones I prefer.
	Although garlic can reduce blood pressure and cholesterol levels for some people, it doesn't work for everyone. It may take up to 3 months to see these effects and the average reduction for cholesterol and blood pressure is about 10%. For people with cholesterol levels of 300 to 400, using garlic alone may not be enough, and other natural or prescription medicines may be required. Cook with garlic for additional benefits.
	Garlic may be effective in killing the H. pylori bacteria often associated with ulcers.
	Garlic can be very useful in eradicating systemic candida infections when used long term.
Cost Factor:	$10-$20
Natural Q:	*Garlic may help lower blood sugars in diabetics.*

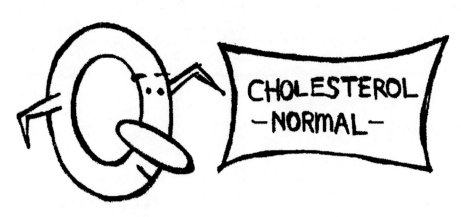

TABLE 12: Ginkgo Biloba

Natural Medicine	Ginkgo Biloba
Use:	Alzheimer's, asthma, depression, peripheral vascular disease, tinnitus, vertigo
Side Effects:	Ginkgo may cause headaches or GI upset.
Drug Interaction:	Ginkgo may thin the blood. Get guidance before using it with Coumadin.
Supplement Interaction:	Ginkgo may interact with natural medicine blood thinners.
Dosage:	Start with 60mg of the extract once daily and work up to 120mg daily in divided doses with food. Some people may require daily doses of 240mg or more in divided doses with food. It may take up to 4 weeks to see full effect of any dose.
Comments:	Ginkgo is a potent natural medicine and should be treated as such. I recommend guidance from a natural medicine expert before starting Ginkgo biloba.
	Ginkgo has been shown to improve altitude sickness.
	Ginkgo is a good choice for diabetic patients since diabetics often have circulatory problems in their legs, eyes, and other organs.
	Ginkgo has been helpful in reducing sexual dysfunction from Prozac, Paxil, or Zoloft in both males and females.
Cost Factor:	$20
Natural Q:	*Ginkgo biloba can be very useful in improving asthma.*

Ginkgo Biloba

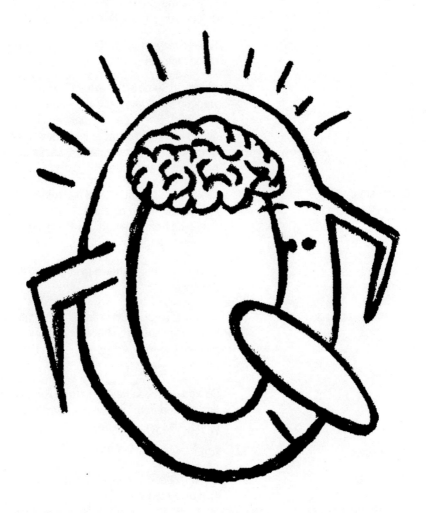

TABLE 13: Glucosamine/Chondroitin

Natural Medicine	Glucosamine/Chondroitin
Use:	arthritis
Side Effects:	Glucosamine/chondroitin may raise blood pressure, blood sugars, and cholesterol levels, but not in every person. May cause GI upset, so take it with food. Both of these natural medicines often come from shellfish sources and in some cases can cause an allergic reaction. If you have an allergic reaction to shellfish that results in difficult breathing, stay clear of these products.
Drug Interaction:	No significant drug interactions with glucosamine. Chondroitin may thin the blood, so use caution in combination with Coumadin, or with aspirin, etc. Monitor for bruising or bleeding.
Supplement Interaction:	No significant supplement interactions with glucosamine. Chondroitin may interact with other natural medicine blood thinners.
Dosage:	Start with 1000mg twice daily with meals for 30 days, then cut back to 1000 to 1500mg daily. Take chondroitin 400 to 1200mg daily in divided doses with meals. It may take up to 90 days or more to see maximum effect, so be patient.
Comments:	Glucosamine and chondroitin are chemically similar and have been shown to increase the production of cartilage and reduce inflammation. The addition of chondroitin may not be necessary, especially if you're on a budget. However, adding MSM to glucosamine can help expedite and improve pain relief. The sulfate form is the preferred form for both glucosamine and chondroitin, even though they may cost slightly more. It's worth it.
Cost Factor:	$20

Natural Medicine	Glucosamine/Chondroitin
Natural Q:	*Using glucosamine sulfate for at least 90 days can significantly improve the pain and reduce the swelling of arthritis.*

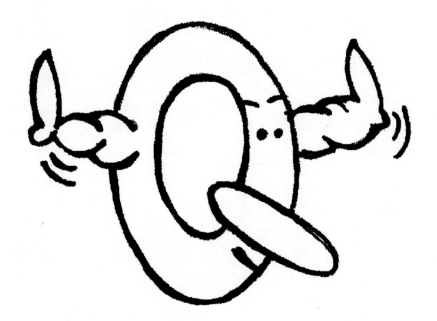

TABLE 14: Inositol

Natural Medicine	Inositol
Use:	ADHD, anxiety, cholesterol, hair growth, insomnia, obsessive-compulsive disorder, panic disorder
Side Effects:	No significant side effects are reported.
Drug Interaction:	No significant side effects are reported.
Supplement Interaction:	No significant supplement interactions are reported.
Dosage:	Start with 500 to 1000mg 1 to 4 times daily as needed for general anxiety. For panic disorder or OCD, work up slowly to 2000 to 3000mg 2 to 4 times daily. Doses up to 18 grams per day (in divided doses) can be used in more severe conditions. Inositol powder is available to help achieve these higher doses.
Comments:	Inositol is in the B vitamin family and sometimes referred to as vitamin B8.
	Inositol can help reduce blood pressure, especially when stress is a factor. It can also help improve symptoms of depression and may help lower blood sugars, as well.
	Because of its low cost and high safety profile, inositol should be considered first line therapy for anxiety.
	Some people become very relaxed using inositol, so use caution before operating heavy machinery, like your car.
Cost Factor:	$10
Natural Q:	*Taking inositol on a regular basis can improve hair growth.*

TABLE 15: Kava

Natural Medicine	Kava
Use:	anxiety , insomnia, muscle spasms, pain, restless legs syndrome
Side Effects:	Kava may cause drowsiness, GI upset.
Drug Interaction:	Kava can cause severe liver problems when used in combination with alcohol or medicines that are hard on the liver, such as acetaminophen (Tylenol), and others. Avoid using kava along with prescription medicines for anxiety, sleep, or depression. This can cause excess drowsiness.
Supplement Interaction:	Kava used in combination with other calming natural medicines like skullcap, hops, chamomile, etc. may cause excess drowsiness.
Dosage:	Start with 70mg of the extract and use it up to 4 times daily as needed. For insomnia, take the dose 30 minutes before you want to go to sleep. Use kava only as needed. Avoid long term, continuous use.

Natural Medicine	Kava
Comments:	Kava can help take the edge off of anxiety without causing that loss of sensorium, but it can still cause drowsiness. Test kava in the safety of your home before operating dangerous machinery, like your car. If you have any history of any liver disorder, stay clear of kava. Kava has a distinctive, pungent taste and smell. There has been a lot of press lately about kava causing liver problems. Kava can be a very safe and effective natural medicine when used correctly. Avoid long-term use or high doses. Do not combine with alcohol. Contrary to logic, kava does not improve the symptoms of Parkinson's, and may make symptoms worse.
Cost Factor:	$20
Natural Q:	*Patients with muscular dystrophy, such as multiple sclerosis, often find relief with kava.*

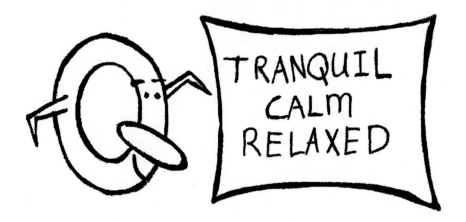

TABLE 16: Magnesium

Natural Medicine	Magnesium
Use:	ADHD, asthma, chronic fatigue syndrome, constipation, diabetes, fibromyalgia, heart palpitations, hypertension, kidney stones, migraines, neuromuscular conditions, PMS, restless legs syndrome.
Side Effects:	Magnesium may cause GI upset, including diarrhea. Too much magnesium may cause muscle weakness.
Drug Interaction:	Similar to calcium, magnesium may interact with the fluoroquinolone antibiotics like Cipro, Levaquin, as well as tetracycline. Take magnesium at least 3 to 4 hours before or after these antibiotics.
Supplement Interaction:	No significant supplement interactions are reported.
Dosage:	Start with 150mg twice daily at breakfast and before bedtime. Some people require doses of up to 1000mg daily, in divided doses with food. It is noteworthy that some people can tolerate large doses without any GI complaints, while others can only tolerate very small doses.

Natural Medicine	Magnesium
Comments:	Many people are magnesium deficient, and this is particularly true as we get older.
	Magnesium should not be taken for long periods without also supplementing with calcium.
	Although it is often rumored otherwise, taking magnesium and calcium at the same time does not seem to significantly change their effectiveness.
	Magnesium, as well as calcium and other minerals like boron, are important in maintaining good bone density.
	Magnesium is important for many bodily functions and can be very useful in relaxing the muscles and the mind prior to bedtime.
	If your kidneys aren't functioning properly, get guidance before you start magnesium.
Cost Factor:	$10
Natural Q:	*Magnesium used with malic acid can improve the muscle pain and tenderness of fibromyalgia.*

TABLE 17: Melatonin

Natural Medicine	Melatonin
Use:	cancer, insomnia, jet lag
Side Effects:	Melatonin may cause drowsiness, but typically not as much as prescription sleeping medicines like Restoril or Ambien. Morning 'hangover' can occur at higher doses. Melatonin can cause headaches and worsen depression in some people.
Drug Interaction:	Although probably safe, I recommend that you don't use melatonin in combination with prescription sleeping medications. Use one or the other. If you've been taking prescription medicines like Restoril, Dalmane, or Ambien every night for a long period of time, don't stop suddenly. Avoid alcohol when taking melatonin.
Supplement Interaction:	Melatonin may cause added drowsiness when combined with natural sleep-inducing medicines like skullcap, chamomile, kava, 5HTP, valerian, and others.
Dosage:	Start with the lowest dose that works and take it 45 minutes before you want to go to sleep. I usually recommend starting with about 0.5mg (1/2mg). Most people require doses of 1 to 3mg when used for sleep, sometimes up to 5mg. Work up to this dose over a period of several weeks. Allow at least 3 to 5 days at a given dose before increasing to the next higher dose. Doses of melatonin for cancer are much higher, often reaching 20 to 40mg daily. Get guidance before you use melatonin for this condition. For jet lag, use 1 to 3mg at bedtime on the day of arrival, and stick with it for 3 to 5 days. When stopping melatonin after long periods of use, taper off gradually.

Natural Medicine	Melatonin
Comments:	Melatonin is a hormone made in our brain. To avoid hormone imbalances, stay clear of melatonin if you're under 40.
	Older patients generally respond very well to melatonin.
	For those who have difficulty falling asleep, use the regular release formulations. For difficulty staying asleep, the sustained release forms may work better.
	Melatonin can be used to help taper off of the benzodiazepine medicines like Valium, Xanax, and Ativan. Get guidance before you attempt this.
	Melatonin is a powerful immune stimulant and antioxidant, and may be useful in treating certain cancers.
	Melatonin may help improve migraine headaches.
Cost Factor:	$10
Natural Q:	*Melatonin can help reduce the symptoms of withdrawal when you stop smoking.*

TABLE 18: Milk Thistle

Natural Medicine	Milk Thistle
Use:	cancer, liver disease of any origin, including cirrhosis and hepatitis
Side Effects:	Milk thistle may cause diarrhea or GI upset.
Drug Interaction:	No significant side effects are reported.
Supplement Interaction:	No significant supplement interactions are reported.
Dosage:	Start with 70mg of the extract twice daily with meals. Sometimes doses of 140mg twice daily or more are used.
Comments:	Milk thistle is part of the ragweed family. Use with caution if you are allergic to daisies.
	Milk thistle has been shown to have antitumor activity and should be considered as part of a natural chemotherapy regimen.
	The liver is responsible for detoxifying our body from the chemicals in the air we breathe and the food we eat, as well as many of the prescription medicines we take. Taking milk thistle on a daily basis may be good preventative medicine. Milk thistle has been shown to help protect, strengthen, and regenerate liver cells.
Cost Factor:	$20
Natural Q:	*Hepatitis C patients report improved energy when they add milk thistle to their regimen.*

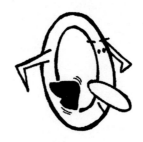

TABLE 19: MSM

Natural Medicine	MSM (methylsulfonylmethane)
Use:	acne, arthritis, asthma, chronic fatigue syndrome, eczema, GERD, hair and nail growth, hay fever, lupus, pain , scars
Side Effects:	MSM may cause GI upset and may keep you awake at night. Don't take MSM past 6pm. Some people experience a detoxification reaction at higher doses. Symptoms of detox include muscle aches, low-grade fever, rash, and headache. This is a sign that MSM is working and usually subsides after several days.
Drug Interaction:	MSM may thin the blood. Use cautiously with medicines like Coumadin, aspirin, etc.
Supplement Interaction:	MSM may cause bruising when used in combination with other natural blood thinners like flax or fish oil, ginger, garlic, ginkgo biloba, and others.
Dosage:	Start with 1000mg daily, and work up to 10,000mg daily in divided doses with meals. Most people see a response at 2000 to 4000mg daily. Take 500mg of vitamin C with each dose to enhance the activity of MSM.

Natural Medicine	MSM (methylsulfonylmethane)
Comments:	MSM is simply organic sulfur and safe to take if you are allergic to sulfa. This sulfur molecule does not cause the 'sulfonamide' type reaction.
	MSM may lower blood sugars in diabetic patients.
	The eye drop formulations of MSM can improve 'bloodshot' eyes.
	MSM is quite effective for skin conditions and can be used both topically and internally for these conditions.
	You may notice increases in your energy level while using MSM, so don't take any within 4 to 5 hours of bedtime.
	MSM can improve cracked and damaged nails, and improve hair growth and fullness.
Cost Factor:	$20
Natural Q:	*MSM may be useful in reducing snoring.*

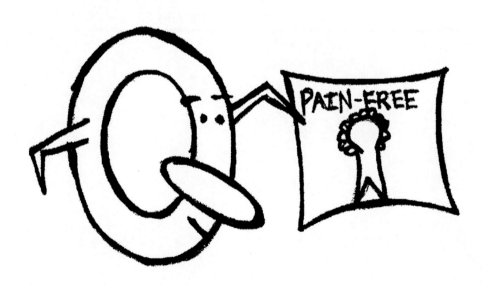

TABLE 20: Progesterone Cream

Natural Medicine	Progesterone Cream
Use:	hot flashes, menopausal symptoms, PMS
Side Effects:	No significant side effects are reported.
Drug Interaction:	No significant side effects are reported.
Supplement Interaction:	No significant supplement interactions are reported.
Dosage:	Rub 1/8 to 1/4 teaspoonful, or about a dime's size, nightly onto your hands, face, thighs, breasts, or stomach. Rotate the application site on a regular basis to avoid skin irritation and cream buildup. Some products have a 'pump' device that can provide a more consistent and accurate dose. Stop using progesterone when your menses begins, and start again when menses is complete. If you're not cycling, take a 5 to 7 day break after each 25 days of continuous use, then begin again. It may take 90 days of continuous use to see maximum effects; however, many women respond within 2 to 3 weeks. Doses can be very individualized, depending on age and physical symptoms, so do get guidance if you're not sure.

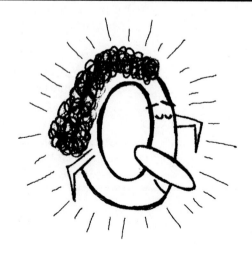

Natural Medicine	Progesterone Cream
Comments:	Progesterone cream is a key component of natural hormone replacement therapy. These products are for topical use, not vaginal use.
	Preparations that contain only wild yam as the active ingredient are generally not effective since wild yam does not convert to progesterone in the human body. Use only products that contain natural progesterone.
	There has been much discussion about whether progesterone cream can help maintain bone density and healthy cholesterol levels like the oral prescription hormones. There is strong evidence that it can. Using progesterone cream as part of a natural hormone replacement regimen can also avoid the increased risk of certain cancers.
	If you're converting from prescription hormones to natural hormone therapy, taper off your prescriptions over time.
	If you have a history of breast or other hormonal cancers, get guidance before you start.
	If you're pregnant or breast feeding, stay clear of progesterone cream.
	If symptoms persist after 3 months of use, talk to your practitioner about testing your saliva hormone levels.
Cost Factor:	$20-$30
Natural Q:	*Supplementing with topical progesterone cream can often improve thyroid function, energy levels, and weight control.*

TABLE 21: SAM-e

Natural Medicine	SAM-e (S-Adenosylmethionine)
Use:	arthritis, depression, fibromyalgia, liver problems.
Side Effects:	SAM-e may cause GI upset. SAM-e may also cause anxiety and flip bipolar patients into a manic state. Do not use SAM-e in bipolar disease.
Drug Interaction:	Do not use SAM-e in combination with prescription antidepressants such as Prozac, Zoloft, Paxil, Elavil, Trazodone, etc.
Supplement Interaction:	Do not use SAM-e in combination with other natural medicine antidepressants such as St. John's wort.
Dosage:	Start with 200mg twice daily on an empty stomach. Most people require 600 to 1200mg daily. Work up to these doses slowly. It can take up to 3 to 4 weeks to see the full effect of any dose.
Comments:	SAM-e stands for S-Adenosylmethionine, an amino acid. Take a B-complex vitamin every day while using SAM-e to prevent the build up of harmful homocysteine levels.
	Store SAM-e in the refrigerator to maintain potency levels.
	SAM-e is expensive; however, it is a good value for people who have osteoarthritis along with depression and/or liver conditions.
	SAM-e can improve bursitis and other painful conditions because of its anti-inflammatory activity.
Cost Factor:	$40
Natural Q:	*SAM-e may be useful for improving memory and easing the symptoms of Alzheimer's.*

TABLE 22: Soy

Natural Medicine	Soy
Use:	cancer, cholesterol, hot flashes, menopausal symptoms, osteoporosis
Side Effects:	Soy may cause GI upset, including nausea and gas. Some people are very sensitive, and even allergic to soy, and may experience rash, itching, and severe GI symptoms.
Drug Interaction:	There is some concern that soy can interfere with proper thyroid function. If you have low thyroid function, use soy sparingly.
Supplement Interaction:	No significant supplement interactions are reported.
Dosage:	Take 25 to 50 grams of soy protein daily. Soy protein shakes come in many flavors. Blend in your favorite fruits and add 1 tablespoonful of flax seed oil for added health benefits. I recommend mixing your soy shakes with soy milk, rice milk, or nut milk, instead of cow's milk. Eating tofu or snacking on soybeans and other soy foods in moderation can also be healthy.
	You can also get the benefits of soy using isoflavone tablets. They contain the active ingredients of soy in tablet form. Take 80 to 100mg of isoflavones daily with food.

Natural Medicine	Soy

Comments:

Although a healthy source of protein, many people are allergic to soy. Try whey or rice protein as alternatives.

Studies show that 25 grams of soy protein daily can not only reduce the risk of breast cancer by about 50% but can reduce the risk of prostate and other cancers, as well.

Soy contains isoflavones, weakly estrogenic plant parts, and, despite controversy, soy may actually reduce (not increase) breast cancer risk in women with breast cancer history.

Cost Factor: $20

Natural Q:

Using a soy, whey, or rice protein shake as a complete breakfast can be a nutritious and delicious way to manage your weight.

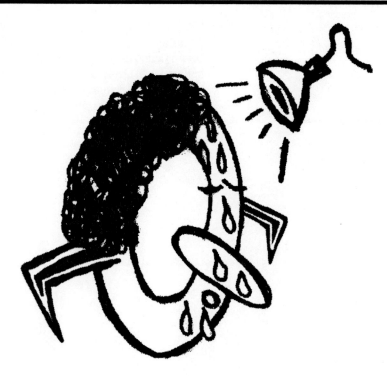

TABLE 23: Spirulina

Natural Medicine	Spirulina
Use:	detoxifier, energy, immune stimulant, weight management
Side Effects:	Spirulina may cause GI upset. Because spirulina is an immune stimulant, it can cause muscle aches, especially in O blood types. Spirulina may cause a 'detox' reaction consisting of muscle aches, skin rash, and a low-grade fever at higher doses. This typically resolves itself over a period of several days.
Drug Interaction:	Although uncommon, the fatty acid content in spirulina may cause blood thinning.
Supplement Interaction:	Spirulina, or other green foods, may increase the potential for bruising or bleeding when combined with other natural medicine blood thinners.
Dosage:	Start with 1 tablet twice daily, 1 hour before meals and work up to 4 to 6 tablets daily, over a period of several weeks. Take spirulina with plenty of water throughout the day. Powdered spirulina can be used to make green drinks or smoothies.

Natural Medicine	Spirulina
Comments:	Spirulina is a complete green food. It is said that one could probably survive indefinitely consuming only spirulina and water.

Spirulina contains high concentrations of green protein, lots of B vitamins, iron, and other minerals.

Spirulina and the other green foods are powerful detoxifiers, and, as such, may initiate a 'detox' reaction. Start slowly.

Spirulina and other greens can help eliminate heavy metal toxins, such as lead, mercury, cadmium, etc. from the body.

Spirulina can be very effective in reducing appetite and managing weight. |
| Cost Factor: | $10 |
| **Natural Q:** | *Spirulina can help lower cholesterol levels.* |

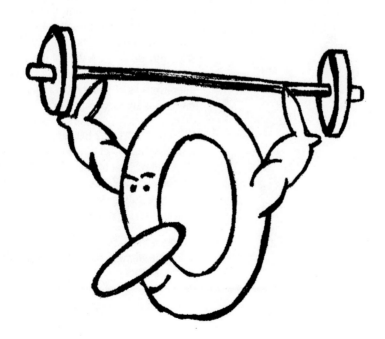

TABLE 24: St. John's Wort

Natural Medicine	St. John's Wort
Use:	anxiety, depression, hepatitis C ,obsessive-compulsive disorder, pain, shingles, wound healing.
Side Effects:	St. John's wort may cause photosensitivity, so wear sunscreen during therapy. St. John's wort may cause irritability, dizziness, and GI upset, and can cause anxiety. Avoid St. John's wort in bipolar disease since it may flip some people into a manic phase. Some people may experience increases in blood pressure and headaches when they eat certain cured foods, white wine, and cheeses, due to their tyramine content. Minimize the consumption of these foods while taking St. John's wort.
Drug Interaction:	St. John's wort has lots of drug interactions. If you're taking any prescription medicines, get guidance before you start. Use St. John's wort with caution if you're taking oral contraceptives (birth control pills) since St. John's wort may decrease estrogen levels, increasing the risk of pregnancy. St. John's wort may decrease levels of the heart medicine digoxin, and may decrease the effectiveness of many prescription antiviral medicines used to treat HIV.
	St. John's wort may thicken the blood, reducing the effect of the blood thinner Coumadin. Do not use St. John's wort in combination with prescription antidepressants like Prozac, Zoloft, Paxil, Elavil, Trazodone, etc.
Supplement Interaction:	Do not use St. John's wort in combination with natural medicine antidepressants such as SAM-e.

Natural Medicine	St. John's Wort
Dosage:	Getting the correct dose of St. John's wort can be tricky, since different manufacturers label their products differently. Start with 1.8mg to 2.7mg of the hypericin extract daily. If you're not sure about the dose in your brand, get some guidance. It may take up to 4 to 5 weeks to see the full antidepressant effect of St. John's wort. When discontinuing therapy, don't stop this medicine suddenly. Instead, taper the dose slowly over several weeks to minimize the withdrawal effect.
Comments:	There is some evidence that people who are blood type O don't respond well to St. John's wort. I recommend reserving St. John's wort for people who are not blood type O, and for those who aren't taking any other prescription medicines.
Cost Factor:	$10-$20
Natural Q:	*St. John's wort salve applied topically can improve the pain and itching of shingle lesions.*

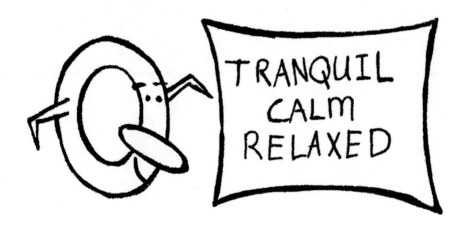

TABLE 25: Vitamin C

Natural Medicine	Vitamin C
Use:	acne, antioxidant, antiviral, arthritis, asthma, cancer, cataracts, glaucoma, hay fever, immune stimulant, lung conditions, memory, varicose veins , wound healing
Side Effects:	Vitamin C can cause GI upset including heartburn and diarrhea, especially at higher doses, and especially when using unbuffered formulations containing straight ascorbic acid.
Drug Interaction:	No significant drug interactions.
Supplement Interaction:	Vitamin C can increase the absorption of iron. If your blood contains too much iron, get guidance before supplementing with vitamin C.
Dosage:	Start with 500mg daily and work up slowly to an average of 1500mg daily in divided doses with food. Some people use doses approaching 20,000mg daily. I prefer the buffered forms of vitamin C, and if your budget permits, the time release forms are nice (but not necessary). Controversy abounds about high dose vitamin C causing thickening of the carotid vessels in some men. If you're a male, and you smoke, get guidance from your practitioner before using high doses of vitamin C.

Natural Medicine	Vitamin C
Comments:	I recommend using vitamin C that is combined with the bioflavonoids, or plant parts, that help enhance the activity of vitamin C. Vitamin C can help reduce the incidence of hay fever allergies and is an important component of any natural anticancer regimen. If you suffer from any eye or skin condition, vitamin C can help improve your condition. If you have weak or fragile blood vessels, vitamin C can help improve their strength and function. Fruits, vegetables, and whole grains are a great dietary source of vitamin C. You've heard it before: 'eat well'.
Cost Factor:	$10
Natural Q:	*Taking 5000mg of vitamin C daily can help repair the lung damage from cigarette smoke and other pollutants, even if you still smoke.*

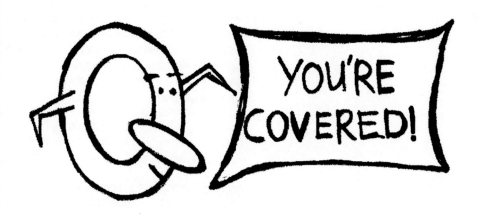

TABLE 26: Vitamin E

Natural Medicine	Vitamin E
Use:	Alzheimer's, antioxidant, asthma, cancer, cataracts, cholesterol, coronary artery disease, fibrocystic disease, leg cramps, lung conditions, memory, menopausal symptoms, neuromuscular conditions , Parkinson's, PMS
Side Effects:	Vitamin E may cause GI upset and headache.
Drug Interaction:	Vitamin E may enhance the blood thinning potential of Coumadin, aspirin, and others. Watch for excess bruising or bleeding, especially with doses above 400 units daily.
Supplement Interaction:	Vitamin E may enhance the potential for bruising or bleeding when combined with natural blood thinners.
Dosage:	Start with 200 units daily with food. This amount can often be found in many high potency multiple vitamins, and is probably enough for most people. Alzheimer's and other conditions may sometimes require doses of 2000 to 3000 units per day. Don't exceed a total of 400 units daily without professional guidance.
Comments:	There is much discussion about natural vitamin E (d alpha tocopherol) versus synthetic vitamin E (dl alpha tocopherol). Vitamin E from natural sources, such as grains or vegetable oils, although a bit more costly, appears to have more activity than the synthetic form, and I prefer it.
	Vitamin E, in combination with vitamin C and other nutrients, is an important part of a natural memory-enhancing regimen.
	Vitamin E is thought to have anti-aging properties and is a powerful antioxidant.

Natural Medicine	Vitamin E
Cost Factor:	$10-$20
Natural Q:	*Applying vitamin E oil to the skin can help heal burns and other skin conditions.*

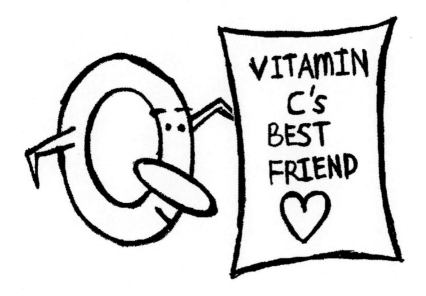

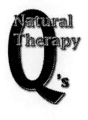

Natural Therapies For Common Conditions

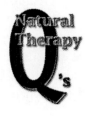

Anxiety

Millions suffer from this disabling condition for a whole host of reasons. If the stress of life is keeping you from true happiness, try something natural.

Take INOSITOL, 500mg up to 2000mg per dose, any time you feel anxious. This medicine is not habit forming; in fact, it's just one of the B vitamins.

Add CALCIUM 300 to 600mg twice daily and MAGNESIUM 200 to 400mg twice daily at breakfast and just before bedtime with a big glass of water. Both of these minerals can help relax the mind and body, and can also improve that restless leg syndrome that many people experience at bedtime.

KAVA is a good back up choice if inositol doesn't quite do the trick for anxiety, or for restless legs syndrome. Follow the label directions on the bottle, and don't exceed the recommended dose. Use kava only for the short term, only if you avoid all alcohol, and only occasionally if you also use Tylenol. If you have any liver problems, stay clear of kava.

Reduce or eliminate sugary foods and drinks (all sodas) from your diet.

Make time to meditate 15 to 30 minutes every day. It's important to connect with your inner self in whichever way feels right to you.

"OM"

Last, and very important, pay attention to the way you breathe. When we tense up, we tend to hold our breath longer, and our breathing can become shallow. This can cause anxiety as well as depression. When you start feeling stressed, try breathing in slowly to a 2 to 4 count, and exhale to a 2 to 4 count. Stay with this breathing technique for at least 5 minutes, or longer. If you begin to feel stressed at work or in a public place, take refuge in the bathroom, or any place where you can be alone for a few minutes. You'll be surprised how good you'll feel when you return to the 'real' world.

Natural Medicine / Technique	Suggested Dosage / Method
INOSITOL	500mg up to 2000mg per dose, any time you feel anxious
CALCIUM	300 to 600mg twice daily
MAGNESIUM	200 to 400mg twice daily at breakfast and just before bedtime with a big glass of water.
KAVA	Follow the label directions on the bottle, and don't exceed the recommended dose.
REDUCE OR ELIMINATE	Sugary foods and drinks.
MEDITATE	15 to 30 minutes every day.
BREATHE SLOWLY	Breathe in slowly to a 2 to 4 count, and exhale to a 2 to 4 count.

Want to reduce your stress levels? See the good in everything and everybody. You'll be surprised at the difference it makes.

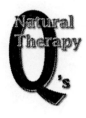

Arthritis

Osteoarthritis is the most common form of arthritis and is caused by a reduction of cartilage, resulting in pain, inflammation, and immobility.

GLUCOSAMINE works well for many people. Start with 1000mg twice daily for about 2 weeks, then reduce that to 750mg twice daily with meals.

Add MSM 1000mg twice daily with meals, along with 500mg of vitamin C with each MSM dose. Stick with this regimen for at least 3 months.

Often, adding those high potency PROTEOLYTIC ENZYMES 2 to 6 tablets 2 to 3 times daily BETWEEN meals can really improve pain and inflammation.

Add 1 tablespoonful of FLAX SEED OIL to your diet once to twice daily with meals. This is especially helpful if you suffer from rheumatoid arthritis.

FISH OIL capsules (1 to 2 capsules twice daily with meals) can also make a big difference. Eating more of your favorite fish every week will also help.

For topical use, try some CAPSAICIN CREAM. This is the active ingredient in cayenne peppers. This substance can help reduce the transmission of pain sensations, but it needs to be used on a regular basis. Apply it to the affected area 3 to 4 times daily for at least 1 week straight.

Reduce the amount of fat in your diet, including dairy and red meat. It's also helpful to cut back on caffeine, tobacco, and sugar consumption, as well as potatoes and tomatoes.

Exercise regularly, even if it's only for short time, or a short distance. Walking is a great way to start.

Natural Medicine / Technique	Suggested Dosage / Method
GLUCOSAMINE	1000mg twice daily for about 2 weeks, then reduce that to 750mg twice daily with meals.
MSM	1000mg twice daily with meals.
VITAMIN C	500mg of vitamin C with each MSM dose.
PROTEOLYTIC ENZYMES	2 to 6 tablets 2 to 3 times daily between meals.
FLAX SEED OIL	Once to twice daily with meals.
FISH OIL	1 to 2 capsules twice daily with food.
CAPSAICIN CREAM	Apply it to the affected area 3 to 4 times daily for at least 1 week straight.
REDUCE FAT	Including dairy and red meat.
REDUCE OR STOP	Caffeine, tobacco, and sugar consumption, as well as potatoes and tomatoes.

Eating pineapple, which contains the enzyme bromelain, as well as sulfur-containing foods like asparagus, eggs, and onions can help improve the symptoms of arthritis.

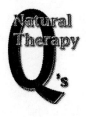

Cholesterol Elevations

High cholesterol plagues millions of people and can contribute to heart disease and stroke. Take a few natural steps to help bring it down.

Taking a GARLIC supplement every day can help reduce cholesterol levels by about 10% in many cases. Take garlic with food, and watch for bruising or bleeding, especially if you're taking other natural or prescription blood thinners.

FLAX SEED OIL can also make a difference. Start with 1 to 2 tablespoonsful daily mixed into a SOY, RICE, OR WHEY PROTEIN SHAKE for breakfast. If you prefer, take it straight, or make a salad dressing with it.

POLICOSANOL, a natural medicine from sugar cane, can also help. Start with 10mg once daily and work up to twice daily, with food. If you're taking Coumadin, or other blood thinners, get guidance before you start.

If results aren't quite where they should be, add NIACIN, vitamin B3, 250mg daily with meals, and work up slowly to 1000mg daily in divided doses. Use the 'flush-free' niacin and insist on the short-acting niacin, rather than the sustained release types. If you have liver problems, get guidance before you start niacin.

Stick with this regimen for at least 90 days before you recheck your cholesterol levels.

Eat lots of fruits and vegetables since these can help bind and eliminate those 'bad fats'. Consume lots of garlic, onions, mushrooms, and whole grains. High fiber diets help reduce cholesterol levels. Try salmon, tuna, or other fish to help put a

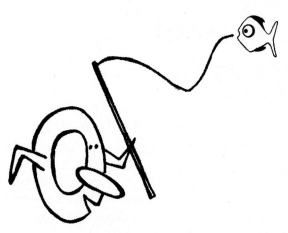

dent in high cholesterol levels. Avoid sweets and sugary foods since these convert to fat. It's also helpful to minimize the amount of dairy and animal protein you consume. Cutting back on fried and processed foods can also make a difference. For best results, cook with olive oil instead of other vegetable oils.

Regular exercise is but another cornerstone for healthy living. Make an effort to develop a regular exercise routine that works for you.

Natural Medicine / Technique	Suggested Dosage / Method
GARLIC SUPPLEMENT	Take garlic with food, and watch for bruising or bleeding, especially if you're taking other natural or prescription blood thinners.
FLAX SEED OIL	1 to 2 tablespoonsful daily mixed into a PROTEIN SHAKE (see below).
SOY, RICE, OR WHEY PROTEIN SHAKE	Once daily at breakfast.
POLICOSANOL	Start with 10mg once daily and work up to twice daily, with food.

Natural Medicine / Technique	Suggested Dosage / Method
NIACIN	250mg daily with meals, and work up slowly to 1000mg daily in divided doses.
INCREASE	Fruits and vegetables (garlic, onions, mushrooms), and whole grains, salmon, tuna, or other fish
AVOID	Sweets and sugary foods
REDUCE	Dairy and animal protein, fried and processed foods.
COOK WITH	Olive Oil.
EXERCISE	Regularly.

Drinking green tea can help reduce your cholesterol levels.

Blue-green algae, spirulina, can also help reduce cholesterol levels. You might also appreciate the side-effects of weight loss and increased energy.

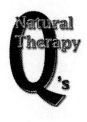

Chronic Fatigue Syndrome/ Fibromyalgia

Here's a condition that is often misdiagnosed and, typically, poorly controlled with prescription medicines. Natural relief is available.

Start with MAGNESIUM 300mg twice daily and MALIC ACID 400mg twice daily with meals.

Add 1 tablespoonful twice daily of FLAX SEED OIL with meals to help reduce any inflammation, balance the immune system, and keep the gut functioning properly.

ALOE VERA JUICE: 1 to 2 tablespoonsful, taken 2 to 4 times daily on an empty stomach can provide additional relief by helping reduce the pain and balancing the immune system.

Adding SAM-e 400mg twice daily on an empty stomach for at least 30 days can also be helpful with both the pain and mood components.

I also encourage the regular and continuous use of ACIDOPHILUS and DIGESTIVE ENZYMES to help improve digestion and utilization of nutrients from your diet. This, along with the aloe vera juice, can reduce the overgrowth of candida in the gut, which, in turn, may be responsible for the symptoms of chronic fatigue and fibromyalgia.

Natural Medicine / Technique	Suggested Dosage / Method
MAGNESIUM	300mg twice daily.
MALIC ACID	400mg twice daily with meals.
FLAX SEED OIL	1 tablespoonful twice daily with meals.
ALOE VERA JUICE	1 to 2 tablespoonsful, taken 2 to 4 times daily on an empty stomach.
SAM-e	400mg twice daily on an empty stomach for at least 30 days.
ACIDOPHILUS	Follow directions on package.
DIGESTIVE ENZYMES	Follow directions on package.

Reducing your consumption of caffeine, sodas, processed foods, and food additives like MSG and aspartame can help improve the symptoms of chronic fatigue.

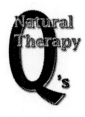

Constipation

Seems simple enough, but many people suffer from chronic constipation. And it's not fun. Why not 'go' natural?

Start with MAGNESIUM 300mg twice daily at breakfast and again at bedtime. I also recommend 1 tablespoonful of FLAX SEED OIL with breakfast every day. For most people, this does the trick.

If you're not quite there, bump the magnesium up to 400mg twice daily, and add 1 tablespoonful 2 to 3 times daily of ALOE VERA JUICE before meals. If diarrhea sets in, adjust your doses down. Your body will let you know what to do, and everyone is different.

Eat lots of veggies, fruits, and whole grains. This will provide the bulk you need to keep things moving, not to mention their nutritious value.

Natural Medicine / Technique	Suggested Dosage / Method
MAGNESIUM	300mg twice daily
FLAX SEED OIL	1 tablespoonful at breakfast daily.
ALOE VERA JUICE	1 tablespoonful 2 to 3 times daily before meals.
INCREASE	Veggies, fruits, and whole grains.

Strive for at least twelve (12) 8-ounce glasses of water every day, from waking until 6pm nightly. Your body will reward you in more ways than one.

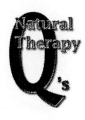

Diabetes

High blood sugars wreak havoc on the human body. Adjusting your diet, bumping up your exercise, and adding a few natural medicines can help you win this battle.

Start with CHROMIUM PICOLINATE 200mcg once to twice daily 45 minutes before you eat, and work up to a maximum of 600mcg daily. This mineral can reduce blood sugars, reduce carbohydrate cravings, and help tone your muscles. If you have kidney problems, get guidance before you start.

The herb GYMNEMA is helpful in reducing blood sugar levels. Start with 200mg daily and work up to 400mg daily, or follow the directions on the bottle you buy.

MAGNESIUM can also lower blood sugars. Start with 200mg twice daily, at breakfast and just before bedtime, and stick with it.

The herb STEVIA is a safe, natural alternative to sugar, aspartame, and others. Not only does stevia not raise blood sugars, it can actually help reduce blood sugars. Try the powder or liquid form the next time you want to sweeten something.

Make sure to monitor your blood sugars more carefully during the first 2 weeks of therapy with natural medicines. It may be necessary to reduce the doses of your other diabetes medications once the natural medicines begin to work, so keep your diabetic doctor in the loop.

Always keep a tube of liquid glucose handy in case blood sugars come down too fast.

Eating the right foods is paramount in improving this condition. Minimize the simple carbohydrates like breads, pasta, candy, chips, and crackers, as well as alcohol and dairy. Focus on eating lots of vegetables, and some fruits. Fruits are high in fiber but are also high in naturally-occurring sugars. Stay away from processed foods, fast foods, fried foods. Consume lots of whole grains, including rice and oats, fish, garlic, onions, and mushrooms. Consume as much fiber as you are able.

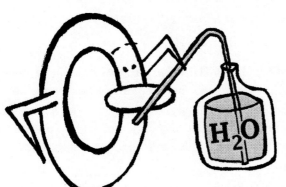

By all means, avoid any foods or beverages that say 'diet', including Sweet'N Low, saccharin, and especially diet sodas. Stick with distilled water or fresh-brewed ice tea with lemon, and a dash of stevia for taste.

Exercise is not only recommended for good health, it can be instrumental in helping reduce high blood sugars. Exercising helps your body push sugar into the cells, where it belongs. Even if all you do is exercise regularly, blood sugars can start to come down.

If you weigh more than you should, make strides toward losing those pounds, but do so slowly, and with realistic expectations.

Natural Medicine / Technique	Suggested Dosage / Method
CHROMIUM PICOLINATE	200mcg once to twice daily 45 minutes before you eat, and work up to a maximum of 600mcg daily.
GYMNEMA	200mg daily and work up to 400mg daily

Natural Medicine / Technique	Suggested Dosage / Method
MAGNESIUM	200mg twice daily, at breakfast and just before bedtime.
STEVIA	Safe, natural alternative to sugar, aspartame, and others.
MONITOR BLOOD	It may be necessary to reduce the doses of your other diabetes medications once the natural medicines begin to work, so keep your diabetic doctor in the loop.
MINIMIZE	Breads, pasta, candy, chips, and crackers, as well as alcohol and dairy.
INCREASE	Vegetables.
EXERCISE	Regularly.

Spirulina can help you lose weight and control your blood sugars. Think green!

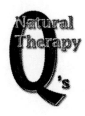

Hypertension

Here's one for the books. Fifty million Americans suffer from high blood pressure. Let's look at some natural ways to help get in control.

Start with CALCIUM 500mg and MAGNESIUM 300mg twice daily with breakfast and just before bedtime.

GARLIC can also put a dent in high pressures. Eat fresh garlic when possible, and supplement with a high quality 'fresh' garlic tablet daily with food.

COQ10 can also lower blood pressures, especially systolic (the 'upper number') pressures. Start with 100mg daily and stick with it. If you take Coumadin, get guidance before you begin.

If stress is a factor, INOSITOL can reduce pressures and stress at the same time. Start with 1000mg 2 to 3 times daily as needed to help you feel more relaxed.

Stay away from processed foods, caffeine, and food additives like aspartame (AKA Nutrasweet) and MSG, and do get regular exercise. Walking 15 to 20 minutes each morning can make a difference.

Natural Medicine / Technique	Suggested Dosage / Method
CALCIUM	500mg twice daily.
MAGNESIUM	300mg twice daily.
GARLIC	Eat fresh garlic when possible, and supplement with a high quality 'fresh' garlic tablet daily with food.
COQ10	Start with 100mg daily and stick with it.
INOSITOL	1000mg 2 to 3 times daily as needed to help you feel more relaxed.
AVOID	Processed foods, caffeine, and food additives like aspartame and MSG.
WALKING	15 to 20 minutes can make a difference.

Meditation is a great way to help lower blood pressure. Why not make it part of your daily routine?

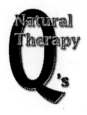

IBS (Irritable Bowel Syndrome)

This one covers a lot of ground, from gas to GERD (esophageal reflux; heartburn). Here are some natural ideas.

Start by using a DIGESTIVE ENZYME with each regular size meal. Take 1 with the first bite of food. If you have ulcers or any GI bleeding, get guidance before you start.

ACIDOPHILUS can also be very helpful. Take 1 to 2 capsules 3 times daily, 1/2 hour before you eat, and stick with it.

ALOE VERA JUICE is a great anti-inflammatory herb and can help reduce GI swelling and pain. Follow the directions on your bottle and take a dose 1 to 3 times daily, 1/2 hour before you eat.

Adding 1 tablespoonful of FLAX SEED OIL once to twice daily with food can help improve the symptoms of IBS. Feel free to mix this with yogurt, cottage cheese, or your favorite beverage to help disguise the nutty oily taste. Some actually enjoy the taste and take it straight. Bon appetit!

PEPPERMINT OIL CAPSULES taken 1 to 3 times daily before meals can bring added benefit. Make sure they're the enteric-coated capsules, not the pure oil.

Consuming lots of fiber is a good idea. Include plenty of whole grains and beans in your diet, and reduce your consumption of alcohol for best results.

Natural Medicine / Technique	Suggested Dosage / Method
DIGESTIVE ENZYME	Take 1 with the first bite of food.
ACIDOPHILUS	Take 1 to 2 capsules 3 times daily, 1/2 hour before you eat.
ALOE VERA JUICE	Follow the directions on your bottle and take a dose 1 to 3 times daily, 1/2 hour before you eat.
FLAX SEED OIL	1 tablespoonful once to twice daily with food
PEPPERMINT OIL CAPSULES	1 to 3 times daily before meals
INCREASE	Whole grains and beans in your diet.
REDUCE	Alcohol consumption.

Avoid wearing tight-fitting clothes or belts around your waist to help reduce the pressure on your GI tract.

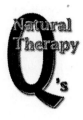

Insomnia

Millions of people are robbed of fulfilling days and lives because they are sleep deprived. Natural relief is available.

Start with CALCIUM 500mg and MAGNESIUM 300mg thirty to 45 minutes before you want to sleep. These minerals can calm the body and mind.

INOSITOL 1000mg just before bed can be added to relax the mind and bring on the sandman.

Many people find improved sleep when they use the hormone MELATONIN. Start with 0.5mg (1/2mg) 45 minutes before you want to go to sleep. You may increase this dose slowly to 3mg over a period of several weeks, if needed. If you fall asleep without trouble but wake during the night, use the sustained release form of melatonin. I don't recommend melatonin under the age of 40, and it should be used only when truly needed. Avoid using melatonin every night, if possible.

Avoid exercising within 6 hours of sleep time, and reduce caffeine and sugar consumption, especially at dinner time.

Fifteen minutes of focused meditation can also help ready your mind for sleep.

Natural Medicine / Technique	Suggested Dosage / Method
CALCIUM	500mg - 30 minutes before sleep.
MAGNESIUM	300mg - 30 minutes before sleep.
INOSITOL	1000mg - 30 minutes before sleep.
MELATONIN	0.5mg (1/2mg) 45 minutes before you want to go to sleep.
AVOID	Exercising within 6 hours of sleep time.
REDUCE	Caffeine and sugar consumption.
MEDITATION	15 to 20 minutes can make a difference.

Reading a book in bed, or playing soft, rhythmic music can help bring you to sleep. Go ahead, give it a try.

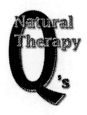

Menopausal Symptoms

Menopausal symptoms are the plague of mature women everywhere. These include hot flashes, mood swings, irritability, insomnia, weight gain, thyroid problems, and more. Natural hormone replacement therapy can be very effective in reducing symptoms and protecting against osteoporosis and cardiovascular problems.

Start with natural PROGESTERONE CREAM. Rub 1/4 teaspoonful or 1 pumpful nightly, into your hands, face, tummy, thighs, or breasts, occasionally rotating sites. Stop for your menses, if you still cycle, and begin again when menses is complete. If you no longer cycle, take a 5 to 7 day break after 25 days of continuous use. Stay with this regimen for at least 90 days.

Drink a SOY PROTEIN shake every day. Add 1 tablespoonful of FLAX SEED OIL and your favorite fruits to the shake and enjoy!

EVENING PRIMROSE OIL capsules have mild estrogenic activity, and they can help improve hormonal symptoms. Start with 1300mg once to twice daily with food.

Take MAGNESIUM 300mg and CALCIUM 500mg twice daily with breakfast and just before bedtime, or with a meal or a snack.

Eating foods high in those natural plant estrogens can also help. These foods include beans, such as garbanzo beans, lentils, green beans, and soybeans. Consume lots of veggies of all kinds, the darker the color the better. Eat generous amounts of fish and whole brown rice, and reduce the amount of red meat and dairy you consume.

Don't forget the water. Drink at least 10 to 12 eight-ounce glasses of water every day to keep your body in good working order.

Walk 15 to 30 minutes or more every day to raise your mood, improve your energy, tone your body, and keep your bones in good shape. You'll be glad you did.

Natural Medicine / Technique	Suggested Dosage / Method
PROGESTERONE CREAM	Rub 1/4 teaspoonful or 1 pumpful nightly, into your hands, face, tummy, thighs, or breasts, occasionally rotating sites.
SOY PROTEIN SHAKE	Once daily with 1 tablespoonful of flax seed oil.
EVENING PRIMROSE OIL	1300mg once to twice daily with food.
MAGNESIUM	300mg twice daily with breakfast and just before bedtime, or with a meal or a snack.
CALCIUM	500mg twice daily with breakfast and just before bedtime, or with a meal or a snack.
INCREASE	Veggies of all kinds, the darker the color the better. Eat generous amounts of fish and whole brown rice.
INCREASE	Garbanzo beans, lentils, green beans, and soybeans.

Natural Medicine / Technique	Suggested Dosage / Method
REDUCE	Red meat and dairy.
WATER	10 to 12 eight-ounce glasses of water every day.
WALKING	15 to 30 minutes or more every day to raise your mood, improve your energy, tone your body, and keep your bones in good shape.

Check your temperature orally 3 times daily, 3 hours apart starting at 10am, for 3 consecutive days. If the average temperature is less than 98.6, you may be hypothyroid. Using progesterone cream can help the body make more active thyroid hormone (T3) and improve your energy, mood, and more.

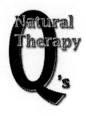

Migraine Headaches

Migraines can totally control your life. Let's explore some natural ideas to help you gain back control.

Start with MAGNESIUM 300mg and CALCIUM 500mg twice daily, at breakfast and just before bedtime. Among other things, it will help you relax and sleep more soundly.

CoQ10 is also an effective way to reduce the pain and frequency of migraines. Try 50mg twice daily with meals.

Add VITAMIN B2, also known as riboflavin, 400mg once daily with breakfast.

Adding 1 tablespoonful of FLAX SEED OIL daily with breakfast can also help improve symptoms.

The herb FEVERFEW has also been used to reduce migraine symptoms; however, I don't like to add it to the regimen until we've tried the above for at least 90 days.

Reduce the number of trigger foods you consume, including simple carbohydrates, alcohol, dairy, tobacco, wheat, corn, food additives and colors, including MSG, processed and aged foods, like lunch meats. It may be wise to do food allergy testing to find out what foods or environmental pollutants you are sensitive to.

Make sure you exercise regularly and enjoy calming music whenever possible. Meditating for 15 to 30 minutes daily, or just taking some special time for yourself every day, can make a difference in your life.

Natural Medicine / Technique	Suggested Dosage / Method
MAGNESIUM	300mg twice daily, at breakfast and just before bedtime.
CALCIUM	500mg twice daily, at breakfast and just before bedtime.
CoQ10	50mg twice daily with meals..
VITAMIN B2	AKA riboflavin, 400mg once daily with breakfast.
FLAX SEED OIL	1 tablespoonful daily with breakfast.
FEVERFEW	If needed, after 90 days of above medicines.
REDUCE	Simple carbohydrates, alcohol, dairy, tobacco, wheat, corn, food additives and colors, including MSG, processed and aged foods, like lunch meats.
EXERCISE	Regularly
MEDITATE	15 to 30 minutes daily,

If you're female and suffer from migraine headaches, hormonal imbalances are often the culprit. Supplementation with topical Progesterone cream could do the trick.

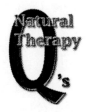

Weight Management

If no diet has ever worked for you, you're not alone. Weight loss and body toning doesn't have to be difficult, expensive, or dangerous. Here are some natural ideas that can really work.

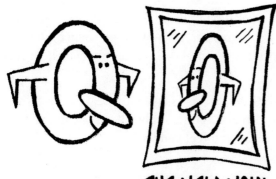

THE NEW YOU!

SPIRULINA, or blue-green algae, does a nice job of reducing food cravings, and it's a great whole-food supplement. Start with 1 tablet 1/2 hour before breakfast and dinner for 7 days, then over a period of 2 weeks, increase your dose to a maximum of 2 tablets 1/2 hour before each meal.

Try a SOY, WHEY, or RICE protein shake as a replacement for breakfast. Stir 1 tablespoonful of FLAX SEED OIL into each serving, blend in your favorite fruits, and enjoy a truly nutritious and satisfying alternative to your usual breakfast.

Many people do very well using a combination of CHROMIUM and GARCINIA CAMBOGIA (also known as hydroxycitric acid, or HCA). These two natural medicines are often found in a combination. But be careful. Many weight products also include stimulants. You don't need stimulants or any other ingredients, so read the labels carefully. Follow the directions on the label, and take your dose at least 1/2 hour before meals. Don't exceed 600mcg of chromium per day. If you have kidney problems, get guidance before you start.

As mentioned, avoid stimulants like Ma Huang (ephedra), guarana, kola nut, and others. These can cause serious medical problems and the results, if any, last only as long as you take the products.

Reduce the amount of simple carbohydrates (sugars) you consume. This includes breads, pastas, cookies, chips. You know the culprits. Minimize processed foods, fast foods, fried foods, and avoid diet sodas, or any food labeled as 'diet'. Consume lean meats and plenty of whole grains, fish, fruits, and vegetables.

Drink plenty of water (you've heard this before, so there must be something to it). Strive for 10 to 16 eight-ounce glasses, or about a gallon per day. Drink 1 to 2 glasses about an hour before each meal.

Exercise doesn't have to be fancy, only regular. Walking or bicycling 15 to 45 minutes 4 to 5 times weekly can make a big difference in the way you feel and look.

Natural Medicine / Technique	Suggested Dosage / Method
SPIRULINA	1 tablet 1/2 hour before breakfast and dinner for 7 days, then over a period of 2 weeks, increase your dose to a maximum of 2 tablets 1/2 hour before each meal.
SOY, WHEY, RICE SHAKE	Replacement for breakfast. Stir 1 tablespoonful of FLAX SEED OIL into each serving.
CHROMIUM and GARCINIA CAMBOGIA (also known as hydroxycitric acid, or HCA)	Many weight products include stimulants with this combination. Don't exceed 600mcg of chromium per day.

Natural Medicine / Technique	Suggested Dosage / Method
REDUCE	Breads, pastas, cookies, chips. You know the culprits. Minimize processed foods, fast foods, fried foods, and avoid diet sodas, or any food labeled as 'diet'.
INCREASE	Lean meats and plenty of whole grains, fish, fruits, and vegetables.
WATER	Drink 1 to 2 glasses about an hour before each meal.
EXERCISE	Walking or bicycling 15 to 45 minutes 4 to 5 times weekly can make a big difference in the way you feel and look.

The key to successful weight management is having realistic expectations. Be patient. If you want to take it off and keep it off, aim for 1 pound of weight loss per week. That's 52 pounds per year!

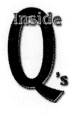

The Inside Q's

So where do we go from here?

Anywhere you want. We've all been blessed with the greatest gift of all: freedom of choice. You can choose the foods you eat, the places you live, the people you marry or live with, the supplements you take. What's more, you can choose how you live, what you think, what you create. Your entire reality is your choice! You create it. If you look at your life and don't like what you see, change it. It's all within your power. And the power is truly within all of us.

Take the time to discover who you are. All you ever wanted to know about yourself is inside of you, and so are the answers to all of your questions, and more. So, how, and where, do you start?

Set aside 30 minutes of your day, every day, just for you. Negotiate this special time with your family or significant other(s), and encourage them to do the same. Find a place in or around your home that makes you feel closer to nature, or to yourself, or what ever feels good to you. Maybe you'll find that special place in your garden, your bedroom, or the park. Just make sure it's a place where you won't be disturbed or distracted.

Turn off your home phone and your cell phone. Take off your watch, close your eyes, and think of nothing. This may sound simple, but it's powerful medicine for your mind, and your body. You'll find it difficult to focus on nothing, since EVERYTHING will want to come into your mind as soon as you quiet it. When thoughts of that deadline, or that phone call you forgot to make come into your mind, refocus.

Start with 5 minutes per day and work up to 30 minutes per day. Take your time. Experiment with it. There is no wrong way, and the results are always positive.

After you've been doing this for a while, you may find that you feel less stressed and that you handle stress, well, with less stress. You may find your blood pressure coming down, your blood sugars may normalize, and all of a sudden you're sleeping better and you have more energy throughout the day. Health concerns may seem to resolve themselves quickly and easily, and you may find that your mood is better than ever. You deserve all of this, and much more.

Many people call this silent exercise, 'meditation'. Call it what you like; just know that when you master this skill, many of the answers you are seeking, in all aspects of your life, will become available to you. We have all the answers. We always have.

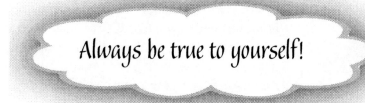

Always be true to yourself!

Printed in the United States
37222LVS00006B/223-270